WHY
KIDS
MAKE
YOU FAT

Also by Mark Macdonald

Body Confidence

**THE PROVEN WEIGHT-LOSS PROGRAM
FOR BUSY PARENTS**

WHY KIDS MAKE YOU FAT

... AND HOW TO GET
YOUR BODY BACK

MARK MACDONALD

Author of the *New York Times* Bestseller *Body Confidence* and Creator of Venice Nutrition

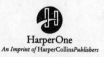

HarperOne
An Imprint of HarperCollinsPublishers

This book is written as a source of information about the effect of foods, vitamins, and dietary supplements on the body. It is based on the research and observations of the author, who is not a medical doctor. The information contained in this book should by no means be considered a substitute for the advice of a qualified medical professional, who should always be consulted before beginning any diet or other health program.

The information in this book has been carefully researched, and all efforts have been made to ensure accuracy as of the date published. Readers, particularly those with existing health problems and those who take prescription medications, are cautioned to consult with a health professional about specific recommendations for supplements, and the appropriate dosages. The author and the publisher expressly disclaim responsibility for any adverse effects arising from the use or application of the information contained in this book.

HarperOne

WHY KIDS MAKE YOU FAT. Copyright © 2015 by Venice Nutrition, LLC. All rights reserved. Printed in the United States of America. No part of this book may be used or reproduced in any manner whatsoever without written permission except in the case of brief quotations embodied in critical articles and reviews. For information address HarperCollins Publishers, 195 Broadway, New York, NY 10007.

HarperCollins books may be purchased for educational, business, or sales promotional use. For information please e-mail the Special Markets Department at SPsales@harpercollins.com.

HarperCollins website: http://www.harpercollins.com

FIRST HARPERCOLLINS PAPERBACK EDITION PUBLISHED IN 2016

Graphics: Vaughan Risher, Venice Nutrition's Director of Graphic Design and Web Development

Recipes: Organized and Overseen by Venice Nutrition's Chef, Valerie Cogswell

Recipe Contributors: Chef Valerie Cogswell, Cashawn McTeer Kirbas, Cassandra Ballon Christie, Kate Flatt, Daniel Miller (aka plant-based man), Shannon Davis, Dawn McGee, Jennifer Fleischer, Paula Lippert, and Rosie Plimpton

Designed by Ralph Fowler
Photograph on page v courtesy of the author.

ISBN 978–0–06–236394–7

Library of Congress Cataloging-in-Publication Data

Macdonald, Mark (Mark Michael).
  Why kids make you fat : and how to get your body back / Mark Macdonald.
     pages cm
  ISBN 978–0–06–236390–9 (hardcover)
  1. Weight loss—Popular works. 2. Detoxification (Health) 3. Exercise. 4. Parenting. 5. Self-care, Health—Popular works. I. Title.
  RM222.2.B647   2012
  613.2'5—dc23   2015009851

16 17 18 19 20   RRD(H)   10 9 8 7 6 5 4 3 2 1

*I dedicate this book to
my three everythings—
my wife, Abbi;
our son, Hunter;
and our baby girl, Hope.*

*Thank you for being my inspiration,
making me laugh, and showing me
how to live life to the fullest.*

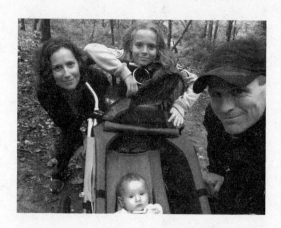

Contents

WHY
KIDS
MAKE
YOU FAT

Introduction

What Happened to the Easy Life?

It was January 2005. My wife, Abbi, was eight months pregnant, and we were super excited to become parents. I was in the best shape of my life, playing tennis five days a week. Abbi and I had unlimited date nights, could go away for the weekend at a drop of a hat, watched the TV shows we enjoyed, and the best part was, we controlled our time. I remember telling Abbi how life would be almost the same when Hunter was born, only better. Of course there would be a few adjustments, but come on, how hard could it be having a kid?

Fast-forward to January 2007 . . . less sleep, less exercise, more unhealthy quick meals, and higher stress. I'm a nutrition and fitness expert, and I was struggling big time with finding the balance of how to be a dad, husband, and businessman and still live a healthy life. Man, it wasn't easy. Now, don't get me wrong. Abbi and I love being parents and have found it to be the most amazing experience of our lives. The main problem was that as Hunter's weight was naturally increasing, so was mine! I remember it like yesterday—one day I woke up, looked in the mirror, thought I was a bit bloated, stepped on the scale, and bam: 235! What?! I'd gained thirty-five pounds in two years.

I had embodied the classic line I heard from my clients: "I know what to do—I'm just not doing it." There was of course some truth to that, but there was more to the story. You see, as my life evolved, my health didn't evolve with it. My tennis time was replaced with changing diapers, my food prep time was replaced with stealing naps, my TV time was replaced with Baby Einstein, and my relaxation time was replaced with constant toy pickup and cleaning. And these were just the lifestyle adjustments *I* had to make—Abbi had twice the responsibilities I had! My point is, there are only twenty-four hours in a day, and the systems and routines Abbi and I had before Hunter were never coming back. We had a simple choice: continue attempting to squeeze parts of our pre-baby life in (at which we were miserably failing), or create new systems and rhythms that would allow us the time to continue being the parents we wanted to be while also creating quality time for each other and for our health.

This is exactly why I've written this book. The honest truth is this: if you don't evolve your health as a parent, your kids will make you fat. Before anyone gets upset, let me clarify that the last thing I want to do is offend you. What I do want to do is have a real conversation. It's not a secret that most of us gain weight and get a bit more flabby as we get older, or that one of the biggest spikes in weight and flabbiness coincides with becoming a parent. This is where we choose to evolve our health and progress, or the regression rapidly begins. As parents, we clearly know it's not our kids' fault we gain unwanted weight and store fat, and it's not an excuse either. It's just a reality. Our kids simply make us rethink our priorities, and we begin to give more to them than to ourselves, which is, of course, natural. The challenge with this mind-set shift is that when you forget about yourself and your health, you can't be the parent or person you used to be, want to be, or are meant to be.

On my desk I have a picture that Abbi and Hunter gave me. It's of Hunter and me playing soccer at a castle in Germany, and the frame reads:

> **Life's Moments . . .** Life is not measured by the number
> of breaths you take, but by the number of moments that
> take your breath away.

In essence, that statement is what this book is all about—not about living healthier but about living better, with a greater quality so you can own those special moments and be the person and parent you want to be. Because without your health, the quality of life you want for yourself and your family is just not possible.

This book will walk you through the evolution that Abbi and I and thousands of fellow parents have gone through to create a healthy life, not just for ourselves but also for our families. I get how busy we all are, so in the spirit of time efficiency, I've written this book as direct and to the point as possible, so it's truly a plug-and-play plan designed to take your body and health to the next level. *Plug-and-play* means the information is presented in a way that makes it easy to understand, quick to implement, and simple to do—exactly what we need as parents.

Now I want to share six quick things with you before you dive in:

- As you already know, I'm a man, husband, and dad, and even though I've coached thousands of women, I grew up with two sisters, and my mom was an ob-gyn (obstetrician/gynecologist) nurse . . . I get that I'm still a man. For this reason, my wife, Abbi, got involved in the making of this book and was a huge help in adding the touch of a female, wife, and mom and in providing a fun spin on how to make it all work as a busy parent. Abbi and I have been together for over twenty years and truly live this plan as a family.

- The engine within this book is the plan. You'll be diving into three phases: Detox, Ignite, and Thrive. Your first eight weeks will be a combination of your Detox, Ignite, and Thrive phases and those eight weeks are called making your 8 Week Run. I fully explain this concept in chapter 2, but until then just know your 8 Week Run is not a running program. Your 8 Week Run is a mind-set that keeps you focused, committed, and pushing hard for a period of eight weeks to break through all obstacles and achieve your health goals.

- As you can see by the title and my introduction, I've written this book for parents, future parents, grandparents, and their family and friends. With that being said, the Detox, Ignite, and Thrive phases work incredibly well for anyone wanting to lose weight and burn fat, regardless of whether or not you're a parent. So dive in and rock the plan wherever you currently sit with your life. It's also important to remember that we each have a different definition of *fat*. Society makes the word *fat* sound negative, but I don't see it like that. When I talk about fat, I simply mean being at a place with your body that you're not happy with—the number on the scale is too high, you feel flabby, your energy is low, your clothes don't fit the way you want them to fit, and so on. Basically, you're not the healthy, lean, and truly confident person you want to be. In literal terms, you just have more body fat than you want. We are all different and have different goals, so I invite you to define what *fat* means to you and, instead of looking at it as a negative word, to strip away all the emotions of how that word makes you feel and focus on the literal term. When you do that, it's no longer an insulting word. It's just a word that means you have some extra body fat to lose. And the reason you want to lose that extra body fat is to look, feel, and be your very best (which is defined by you).

- As I shared, my goal with this book is for it to be a completely plug-and-play program. For this reason, there are some details I won't be discussing, like the types of metabolism, goal setting, in-depth meal plans, the science of exercise, and so on. I covered all of that info in my *New York Times* bestselling book *Body Confidence*. Please refer to *Body Confidence* for more detailed information. *Body Confidence* is an excellent read after this book, and it will help you continue Thriving with your plan.

- The plan presented in this book is designed to help you lose weight, burn fat, increase energy, and permanently reprogram your metabolism. I also know that about 3 percent of the population wants to gain weight. Now, I get that's a foreign concept to most of us, but hey, 3 percent correlates to millions of people and many are parents, so it's important to have a solution for them too. If that's you or if your goal is to simply become healthier and not lose weight, the plan will still work incredibly well for you. You may just need to increase your portion sizes based on your goal. I suggest reading this book along with *Body Confidence* and focusing on the goal type 2 meal parameters presented in chapter 5 of *Body Confidence,* in which the nutrition recommendations are designed to help people gain weight. This is also a great solution for any kids who are athletes and/or want to gain weight.

- Finally, as a coach, I've clearly seen how the success stories of others provide us with the inspirational fuel to see the possibilities we can have with our own health and quality of life. For this reason, I've sprinkled the book with motivating stories and before and after photos from fellow busy parents walking a path similar to yours. Seeing their success and reading their stories will motivate you to stay the course and help you to build momentum as you begin to live your plan.

Okay, it's game time. Once and for all, the dieting madness stops! It's time you learn how to permanently lose your bloat, melt your belly, and live your life. Always remember the transformation starts with you! Next level, here we come . . .

> ## ► Quick Support Note

It's extremely important to have support every step of the way as you live your plan and make your 8 Week Run. For this reason we've created a powerful community of people just like you, taking their body and health to the next level. To join the community and share ideas, exchange recipes, and inspire one another every step of the way, simply visit *www.WhyKidsMakeYouFat.com/ Community* and be part of the experience.

1% at a Time . . . It's All About Baby Steps

I remember being seven years old in the living room of our house and asking my mom for a banana. I stood there for about a minute repeatedly asking her, and she kept gently replying "What do you need, Mark?" Every time I asked and couldn't get an answer, my frustration grew, eventually to the point of a full-scale meltdown complete with tears. In my mind what I was asking for was so clear, but my mom and everyone else in the world couldn't understand my words.

You see, I had a severe speech impediment that made it difficult for me to form words. My mom, dad, teachers, and I thought I would outgrow it, but by the time I was seven, things seemed only to be getting worse—I couldn't even say my own name. It's funny how we remember things from our childhood. I can vividly remember feeling like an outsider who couldn't communicate with people. I was frustrated with the world at seven, not even really knowing what that meant. I kept hoping that I would miraculously get better, not be slow in school. I wanted to excel like my friends did, but that just wasn't happening.

At the end of first grade, my teacher, Mrs. Painter, had a meeting with my parents and wanted me to repeat first grade due to my challenges with speech. Mrs. Painter was a terrific teacher who really cared about my success, and she was concerned that I was falling too far behind. When my parents came back from the meeting, they shared what Mrs. Painter had suggested, and it crushed me. I felt like a failure. I didn't want to be different, and I didn't want to be made fun of anymore—I just wanted to be normal.

My mom asked me what I wanted to do. I told her that I needed to get to second grade and that I would do anything it took to get there. She smiled and said, "Then let's find a way." My mom called Mrs. Painter, told her that I was going to move on to second grade, and asked for a referral to the best speech therapist in the school system. My mom then looked at me and provided me with my motto for the rest of my life (even though neither of us knew it at the time). She said, "Mark, this isn't going to be easy. It's going to take a lot of work, and it doesn't matter how quickly your speech improves. All that matters is it improves, 1 percent at a time."

It took me three years of daily work, endless hours of speech practice, but by fifth grade I was communicating, excelling, and loving the world. My mom and my dad and my incredible speech therapist, Mrs. Lathrop, all focused on 1 percent improvement at a time, which was our motto for three years. No matter how frustrating things got or how much it felt at times that my speech would never improve, slowly and steadily, 1 percent at a time, it progressed . . . until finally I was there.

Since I was seven years old, 1 percent has been my motto. I've lived it and seen its power—as a child learning how to speak, as an athlete earning a college scholarship, as a husband growing in a relationship, as a father seeing his child flourish, and as a coach working with thousands of clients to help them let go of the quick-fix dieting madness and permanently reprogram their metabolism.

I'm assuming that if you're a parent, you would share the same advice with your children as my mom did with me. We teach our kids to pace themselves, to understand that results can't come overnight, and that it takes consistency to truly achieve greatness. The challenge (and I'm guilty of it too) is that sometimes we forget that advice ourselves, especially with unwanted weight gain. As I shared in the introduction, that happened to me from 2005 to 2007 when I became frustrated that I'd gained thirty-five pounds as a new dad. The frustration I felt is what countless parents feel every day.

That frustration is what triggers the desire for immediate results, wanting to do whatever it takes to drop weight, fit into pre-baby clothes, and just not be so tired (especially with a newborn!). Think back to anything you've excelled at in life. Was it achieved overnight, or was it accomplished through 1 percent improvements? I love using the analogy of baby steps. Each step a baby takes represents months of hard work in the making, leading up to that moment of breaking through and actually walking.

That's why your first action item as you take on this plan and prepare to make your 8 Week Run is to shift your mind-set to 1 percent. It is designed to start you on the right path, help you begin to gain confidence, and give you results. Imagine if you improve one thing about your health per day for the next 365 days—within a year either your goals will be achieved or you'll be on a steady course to achieving them. The reality is that your health is dynamic and your body is constantly changing, so whether you notice it or not, you are either moving forward or moving backward. But as long as you're aware and are taking steps 1 percent at a time, you are always moving forward.

As you begin to shift your mind-set to 1 percent improvements, there are two additional coaching strategies to keep your mind-set locked in on 1 percent. First, your actions must match your expectations. Second, you need to be clear on your mode.

Your Actions Must Match Your Expectations

My client Ivette Montilla had three kids and always wanted to drop her excess weight. She would set her goals (expectations) super high, be rock solid on plan for two weeks, and then life would push back (raising three kids does that to you), her actions (effort) would slip, and she would go back to her old eating and exercise habits and quit the plan. Ivette and I had many conversations about how she continually set herself up to fail, about how the life she lived before being married and having children was not the same as her current life. She desperately wanted her pre-baby body back, and I told her she could once again be that lean, mean, fighting machine—she just needed to shift her mind-set and make sure her actions matched her expectations. Basically, Ivette needed to adjust the timeline of her goals to match what was realistic for her to do. She took the coaching, dropped twenty-seven pounds and seventeen inches, and got her pre-baby body back in eight weeks.

Ivette Montilla

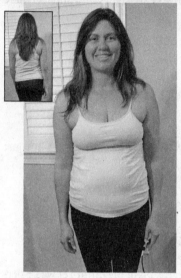

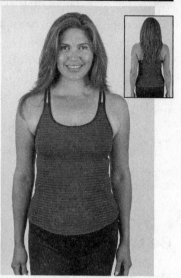

before

after 8 weeks

Ivette Montilla and her kids

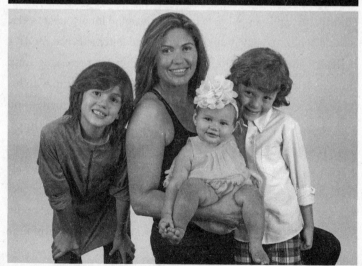

beyond 8 weeks

As you make your 8 Week Run be sure your actions (effort) match your expectations (goals). If you are struggling and feel there is a disconnect, you have two options:

- Raise your actions (effort) to match your expectations (goals)

- Lower your expectations (goals) to match your actions (effort)

Remember, it's not how fast you cross the finish line—it's just important that you cross it!

Be Clear on Your Mode

My friend Rob was doing great on his plan, his mind-set was 1 percent, and his actions matched his expectations. But as we all know as parents, life continually shows up (unforeseen circumstances), and that happened to Rob. One of his boys had complications with appendicitis and was going to be in the hospital for a couple weeks. Rob had to immediately shift his goals and enter survival mode—basically doing everything he could to prevent regressing until things settled down a bit and he could get back in rhythm with his food and exercise. Rob made the adjustment, his son got better, and within a few weeks, he was rocking his plan and back in rhythm.

This is what being clear on your mode means. As you make your 8 Week Run, life may show up, but that doesn't mean you quit your plan . . . no way! You keep moving forward; you just make the necessary adjustments based on your mode. Here are the three modes and examples of where each mode falls in the spectrum within the flow of life:

- **All-in mode:** This is what your 8 Week Run is all about—
  detoxing your body and igniting your metabolism to get
  fast and safe results. You're typically in all-in mode at the
  beginning of the new year, two months before summer, a few
  weeks before a big event, in preparation for a beach vacation,
  or when reading this book for the first time! Basically, you
  shift into this mode when you're highly motivated to go for
  it big time with your food and exercise. This is when you eat
  extra clean and train at a super-intense level.

- **Progression mode:** Your daily routine, a level of
  consistency in your week, or a sense of calmness in your
  life are fantastic examples of when your goal should be
  steady progress that brings steady results. This is your most
  important mode because it's the one that truly will set you
  up with permanent results and will develop powerful food
  and exercise rhythms to look and feel your best. This mode is
  your Thrive phase, week nine and beyond of your plan, and
  is designed specifically for you to use after your 8 Week Run.

- **Survival mode:** During the holidays, a family emergency,
  a major work deadline or trip, a vacation, or a move into a
  new house are all perfect examples of when your goal should
  be to simply maintain your weight. Basically, you shift into
  survival mode and do just enough to prevent regressing. We
  think we must always be progressing with our health goals,
  but the reality is, many times just surviving is a victory
  in itself.

One quick, important thing to remember is that whatever mode
you're in, everyone lives at different levels within each mode. There

is no race with your results. Keep reminding yourself of the lesson my mom taught me when I was seven—it's all about 1 percent and taking those baby steps. It's amazing to see the compound effect of what a 1 percent effort can yield!

Okay, your action items for this chapter are set. Here's a recap and a suggestion for each:

Know It's All About a 1% Mind-Set

- Write down at least one thing you will improve each day with your plan to ensure at least 1 percent progress.

Make Sure Your Actions Match Your Expectations

- Each week evaluate your results and effort to make sure they are connected.

Be Clear on Your Mode

- Define the mode you're in (you should be getting primed for all-in mode because it's 8 Week Run time) and evaluate your mode every two weeks to ensure all is aligned.

Your mind-set is dialed in, so get ready—it's time to make your 8 Week Run!

Making Your
8 Week Run

Life is all about making runs—from growth spurts, to big homework projects, to studying for final exams, to preparing for a wedding, to buying a house, to making it through the first three months with a newborn, to working late to meet a deadline, to writing a book, to clearing your schedule to enjoy the holidays, to losing weight for a vacation. Basically, almost everything we do has moments of pressure and pushing hard (your run) followed by moments of calmness and consistency (your recovery). Our body and mind are designed this way, which is exactly why dieting is so exciting. Dieting fits perfectly into the idea of making a run. The problem with dieting is that most of the weight loss achieved during the run is gained back during the recovery. This is caused by two factors:

- The diet is based on deprivation (typically calorie and/or carbohydrate restriction).

- The diet isn't something you can or want to make a way of life.

I get that success breeds success and that when taking on your health, building momentum out of the gate is crucial, which is exactly why dieting is so appealing. This is even more true as parents, as our schedules can become chaotic and unpredictable at any given time. A simple phone call from the school about a sick child causes your perfectly planned day to be immediately derailed. This amps up your need for quick results even more, wanting to steal that time and at least feel progress for a moment. But what's the point if your success disappears after you make your run? You then have to start another run, chasing the same goal you had already achieved but couldn't maintain, and never truly moving forward.

This is exactly the challenge Gina Nassar experienced for many years. As a busy mom, Gina was always looking for the perfect diet to help her shed weight quickly. Gina had lost forty pounds ten times, and she loved the fast results from dieting but hated the yo-yo effect it caused. Every pound Gina would lose would quickly come back, and with each new diet she tried, the weight would be harder to drop. Gina was searching for something that would give her the momentum she needed and at the same time set her up to win long term so the pounds she lost would stay off permanently.

This is what making your 8 Week Run is all about—getting your dieting fix without actually dieting. Sure, the weight comes off quickly, but it comes off the right way, not by starving yourself, cutting carbs, or doing endless hours of exercise. Gina made her 8 Week Run and lost twenty-two pounds and eighteen inches, but

Gina Nassar

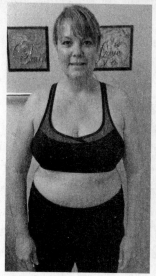
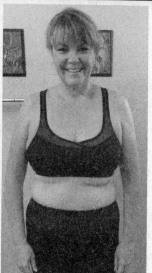

before   after 8 weeks

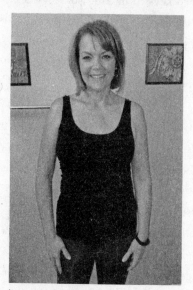

beyond 8 weeks

what's even more impressive is that as she lived her Thrive phase, the pounds and inches kept dropping. Eight months later (her 8 Week Run plus six months of Thriving), Gina had dropped forty-five pounds and thirty-four inches and had truly evolved her plan into a way of life for herself and her family. Now she never needs to worry about the dreaded forty pounds coming back; she knows exactly how to keep them off.

Just like Gina experienced, imagine making a run that delivers the same fast results you get from dieting but is designed to set you up to win long term. A run that is simple to understand and easy to do. A run that builds momentum each week and turns your body into a fat-burning machine. A run that actually leads you into making your food and exercise a way of life and reprograms your metabolism. Now that's a run we all want to make, and that's exactly what your 8 Week Run is all about!

There are two keys to making your 8 Week Run: first, knowing your food is your foundation, and second, mastering the three phases of your plan.

Food Is Your Foundation

As parents we always think to ourselves that we can exercise off the pounds—it just seems easier than dialing in on our food. Plus it makes us feel better to think we can eat our favorite foods and then just burn off those calories with some extra activity. Please don't shoot the messenger, but I have bad news for you and every parent in this world: *there's no workout that can outwork a bad diet.* I know that's tough to hear.

Now don't get me wrong. Exercise is an important piece in your 8 Week Run—it's just not your foundation. Look at exercise as the piece in your plan that burns your fat, builds your muscle, and ignites your metabolism when your food is right. Many people think dieting is the way to get their food right, but unfortunately all dieting does is create calorie and carb deficits that eventually lower your energy, increase your cravings, burn your muscle, and make you crack. And when I say "crack" that's exactly what we've all done when we reach for those doughnuts, pizza, candy, ice cream, cookies, and so on. You dive into whatever foods you love and crave like you haven't eaten them for years. This then makes you bloated, stores fat, and leaves you feeling frustrated that you cracked.

The good news is, there's a reason we crack and better yet, a solution. Those moments of cracking are caused by calorie and carb deficits and unbalanced blood sugar. The truth is, your food should never be used to just lose weight—your food should be used to create hormonal balance in your body. This creates an internal environment where you lose weight without deficits and, most importantly, you keep the weight off as well as prevent cracking! It's simple to do, and I'll teach you how by eating in threes.

Eating in threes balances your blood sugar, protects your muscle, and triggers your body to consistently release stored fat. Eating in threes is eating every three hours with the right balance of protein, fat, and carbohydrates. Eating protein positively affects your blood sugar hormone glucagon (raises your blood sugar), eating carbs affects your blood sugar hormone insulin (lowers your blood sugar), and eating fat slows down the rate of digestion by inhibiting the release of HCL (your stomachs acid). The combination of the three nutrients in the right portion sizes and intervals keeps your blood sugar balanced.

Your entire 8 Week Run is centered on eating in threes. Here are two graphics, the first showing why you need to eat in threes to

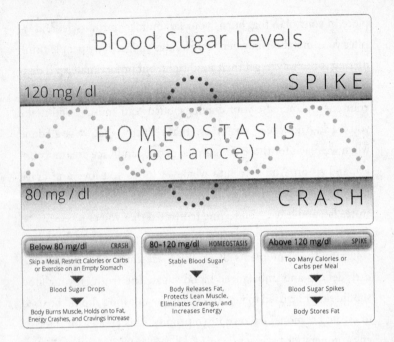

keep your blood sugar balanced and what happens when it spikes or crashes.

And the second graphic (on the opposite page) is a simple but effective visual of what eating in threes actually looks like on your plate. Your protein, carb, and fat choices are presented in the next few chapters, as well as your portion sizes, so no need to imagine what they are now—just make sure to understand the concept and visually connect to the graphic.

Three Phases of Your Plan

The three phases of your plan are designed to deliver fast results and keep momentum flowing while also leading you into a way of life. Phase 1: Detox will cleanse your body to lose your bloat (water

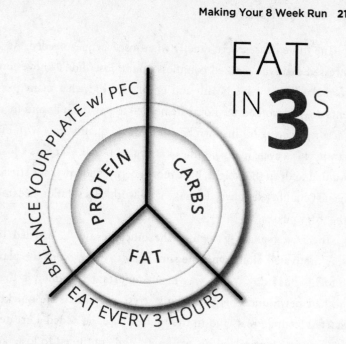

EAT
IN **3**s

retention). Phase 2: Ignite will help your body to burn fat and melt your belly. Phase 3: Thrive will reprogram your metabolism so you can live your plan with your family and friends.

The next three chapters fully dive into each phase and set you up with a plug-and-play plan that's easy to understand, quick to implement, and simple to follow. Here's a snapshot of each phase:

Phase 1: Detox

Lose Your Bloat (Week 1)—Cut, Clean, Flush

Phase 2: Ignite

Melt Your Belly (Weeks 2–4)—Burn, Sculpt, Restore

Phase 3: Thrive

Live Your Life (Weeks 5–8 and Beyond)—Reprogram, Diversify, Energize

The three phases were exactly what Jose Vazquez needed. As a stressed dad who worked countless hours, Jose didn't know how to make time for his health and family. He did what many parents do—he worked the hours he needed to pay the bills and then sacrificed caring for his own health to spend quality time with his family. It's a cycle many families know oh too well. Of course, Jose wanted to drop the weight, have more energy, and lower his stress; he just couldn't see a way to make it all work. His solution became the three phases.

The Detox phase gave him the quick results he needed to stay motivated along with the simplicity to easily work the plan into his busy day. What was most important to him was that he had newfound energy and his stress decreased. He quickly started feeling great, and in the Ignite phase, he added a greater food variety, optimized his workouts, and continued to lose fat, pounds, and inches. The Thrive phase allowed Jose to take his eight weeks of progress and shift his new plan into a way of life by reprogramming his metabolism, diversifying his food and exercise, and including his family and friends. In just eight weeks, Jose lost twenty-nine pounds, twenty-four inches, and two pants sizes. And the fun didn't stop there. Jose kept losing pounds and inches. With this program, Jose was finally able to balance his health, work, and family life while efficiently managing his stress. Just look at his beyond eight weeks photo showing him lean, muscular, and confident!

Jose Vazquez

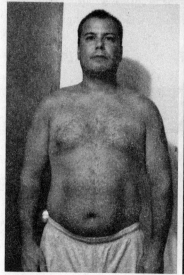 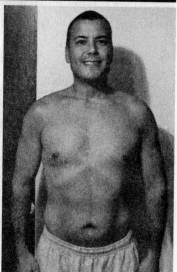

before   after 8 weeks

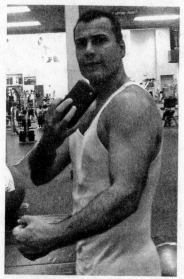

beyond 8 weeks

Okay, now you're prepped, feeling the motivation, and ready to take action! It's time for eight weeks of pushing hard, having fun, and unlocking your body's full potential. Get your engines revved up . . . it's Detox time!

> ## Important Action Items Before You Make Your 8 Week Run

Your weight is only part of the equation to your overall health success. Your weight will make big drops and then recalibrate and drop again—it's just how your body works. Before you start your 8 Week Run, record your baselines for multiple progress markers. This ensures you set yourself up to win and keeps you focused on much more than just weight. Here are five markers to start with:

- **Weight:** Before you begin, weigh yourself once first thing in the morning and record your starting weight. Then wait to weigh again until after your Detox phase (one week). *Only weigh yourself once a week throughout the 8 Week Run, always first thing in the morning.*

- **Inches:** Measure your chest, arms, waist, hips, and thighs and record your starting measurements. Weight might hold at moments, but inches will keep dropping.

- **Body fat percentage:** After you drop your bloat (water retention) in your Detox phase, you want to make sure additional weight loss is all fat and you maintain or increase your lean body mass (mostly muscle). You can get your body fat measured at any local health facility, or you can purchase a body fat scale online or in a store (Tanita makes great quality body fat scales).

- **Before and after pictures:** A picture is worth a thousand words. Countless times my clients have skipped taking a before picture because they didn't want to really see what they looked like, only to wish later that they would have taken one. I get that we're all shy at times, but take one, even if you keep it to yourself. Chances are, once you have your after picture, you'll love to show your before picture! I also suggest taking weekly pictures—front, back, and side—to really see the difference each week. Trust me on this. I can share that every person with a before and after picture you see in this book felt just like you, a bit hesitant at first about snapping a before picture, but now, they are all so happy with their results that they had the courage to share that before picture. A before picture is more than a start for you; it's a statement saying, "No more. I'm ready to take action."

- **Energy:** After your first couple days, your energy will be increasing by the day. Rate your energy 1 through 10, 1 being the lowest and 10 being the highest. Then each week you can see if that number is improving. This lets you stay in touch with how your body is feeling internally as well as how it's looking externally.

➤ **Quick Info and Support Tip**

As you make your 8 Week Run and expand your boundaries, you'll have more questions and will be looking for additional ideas on how to continue maximizing your Detox, Ignite, and Thrive phases. For this exact reason, there are blogs, webinars, coaching videos, and much more available for you by visiting *www.WhyKidsMakeYouFat.com/8weekrun.* The site is designed to build off the themes in this book and *Body Confidence* to provide you with not only information but also guidance to help keep your plan simple, fun, and realistic.

3

DETOX:
Lose Your Bloat

Week 1: Cut, Clean, Flush

I love watching kids take on new adventures. The younger they are, the more fearless they are. Whatever the task, they're all in, not worrying about the outcome. As they enter first grade and beyond, a piece of that fearlessness leaves and they begin to care more about excelling at their tasks. For my son, Hunter, the things he understands quickly and naturally does well pique his interest, which drives him to work harder at fine-tuning those skills—whether it's juggling a soccer ball, throwing a football, riding a bike, acting in a play, reading a book, or putting a puzzle together. The things he doesn't think he does well enough, or that don't click with him, lose his interest.

The reality is, that's just human nature. We all like learning new things, but as we expand our boundaries, we also need progress to justify the effort and feel it's worth our time. Through all my years of coaching clients, this statement resonates deepest in explaining why immediate progress in anything you do is crucial from the start:

> Progress fuels motivation, motivation builds momentum, momentum creates consistency, consistency inspires confidence, confidence delivers results, and results drive lasting change.

As parents, it's not easy to live this flow. We each experience moments of it, but since being a parent is a twenty-four-hour-a-day job, something always seems to disrupt the pattern. That's exactly why week one of your 8 Week Run is specifically designed to deliver maximum results and explode you out of the gate.

You see, most of us are living at an inflated weight, a weight that is made up of at least five to ten pounds of additional bloat (water retention). Think back to a time when you ate better, drank more water, and engaged in some exercise . . . most likely you dropped a few pounds really quickly. That quick weight loss is part of the excess bloat your body holds from living a busy and hectic life. Lack of sleep, daily stress, processed foods, and not drinking enough water are all contributors to holding that extra bloat.

Detoxes and cleanses are so popular because of the inflated weight most of us have. The challenge with most detoxes and cleanses is that they're designed as a diet and short-term fix to a long-term problem. Losing your inflated weight isn't your challenge; I'm assuming you've lost that first ten pounds many times in your dieting history. Most have. The real challenge is how to detox and cleanse effectively while evolving into a plan you can actually make a way of life. Without that evolution, all the weight you lose will just come back a month or two after the detox.

Your seven-day detox plan will trigger immediate weight loss that you'll clearly see and feel. The average weight loss in the Detox phase is seven to ten pounds. This instant weight loss progress becomes inspiration that awakens confidence and belief in what is possible with your body. The power that week one will provide you with will become the motivational fuel to burst you into your Ignite phase (weeks two through eight).

This is exactly what Michelle Totten needed as she started her 8 Week Run. Michelle had just had her third child and was struggling to lose her baby weight. With her first two kids, the weight seemed to drop off with ease, but not this time. What used to work for Michelle wasn't working anymore. She realized she was a bit older, had more demands and distractions, and thought maybe those two factors, along with this being her third pregnancy, were making her baby pounds harder to shed this time around. Regardless, she wanted the weight off fast, but also safely. With a newborn and two other kids, Michelle needed lots of energy and a plan that would work for her and that would allow her to easily integrate what she was eating into meals for her husband, Scott, and their family. Michelle made her 8 Week Run and dropped twenty-eight pounds and twenty-three inches in eight weeks. As she entered her Thrive phase, she dropped another ten pounds!

Michelle shared with me that the fuel that sparked her momentum was the Detox phase. The powerful results she saw and felt that first week gave her the confidence and motivation to accelerate into her Ignite phase. In addition, Michelle's actions inspired her husband, Scott, to join in on the fun. When Scott made his 8 Week Run,

Michelle Totten

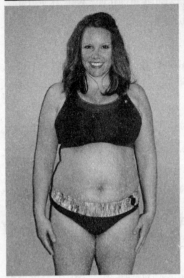

before

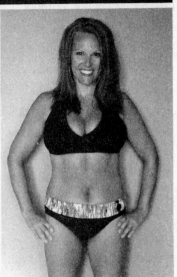

after 8 weeks

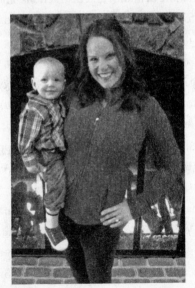

beyond 8 weeks

Scott Totten

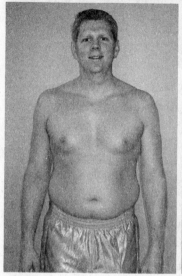

before

after 8 weeks

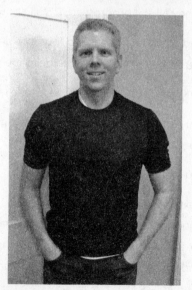

beyond 8 weeks

he dropped thirty-one pounds and seventeen inches, and he has lost another ten pounds as he's living his Thrive phase with Michelle.

➤ Quick Detox Weight-Loss Tip

Now that you're inspired by Michelle and Scott's results, here is some information to help prepare you for your Detox phase:

- Your weight loss in the Detox phase depends on the speed of your metabolism and the amount of inflated weight you have. The average weight loss your first week is seven to ten pounds. Some people drop more than ten pounds, and some people drop less than seven pounds. The important thing to remember is that regardless of the amount of weight each person lost, they all still progressed. It's all about 1 percent.

- Extend your Detox phase to fourteen days (instead of seven) if one or more of these describe you:

  — You have fifty pounds or more to lose

  — You currently drink alcoholic beverages three or more times per week

  — You are a smoker

- You extend your Detox phase because, under these conditions, it may take longer than seven days to detox and prepare your body for the Ignite phase. This extended detox will help maximize your body's fat-burning ability.

Three Steps to Detox: Cut, Clean, Flush

Your Detox phase loses your bloat as easy as 1, 2, 3:

Step 1: Cut

Step 2: Clean

Step 3: Flush

You cut the foods that bloat you, you add the clean foods to cleanse, and you flush the toxins with H_2O.

Step 1: Cut

Detoxing is all about cleaning out your system. Imagine getting an oil change for your car but only adding new oil and still using your old, dirty, and used-up oil filter. As fresh and high quality as that new oil is, it still will be processed through that old filter. This means your car's engine is still getting a lot of grime and grit from the old filter and losing the benefit of the new oil so it won't run as well as it could be running. This concept parallels perfectly with your body. Eating cleaner without detoxing is just like getting an oil change without changing your filter. It only solves part of the problem, so to maximize the cleaner foods you're eating, you also need to clean up your body's filters by removing all the gunk, which will get your metabolism running like a well-oiled machine!

As you detox, you'll also be losing excess bloat. Bloating slows down the speed of your metabolism, inflates your weight, and makes your clothes feel a size too small.

It's time to get you comfortably fitting back into your pre-baby jeans (this is true for both men and women) and lose that muffin top, aka love handles. To do that, your first step is to cut the foods and drinks that cause bloating. Below is a list of foods that make you retain water, followed by a short explanation as to why each food or drink should be removed in this phase.

> ### ➤ Quick Tip
>
> Before you start cursing me, I promise you'll be able to bring these foods moderately back into your meal plan if you so desire, during your Thrive phase, and a few during your Ignite phase.

Foods to Cut During Your Detox Phase

Gluten

Gluten is a hot topic and is quickly being recognized as one of the biggest bloating and inflammatory ingredients in foods. Gluten is a complex protein that gives bread its elasticity and is extremely hard for your body to digest. It's typically found in most bread products, pastas, and cereals. This difficulty with digestion is what leads to inflammation and bloating. Look for gluten-free labels.

Soy

Soybeans contain organic compounds called isoflavones. These compounds trigger your body to produce the hormone estrogen, and estrogen causes your body to store fat and bloat. Estrogen is an important hormone in women and men (that's right—men have a little estrogen too!). The challenge with estrogen is when your body produces too much, which is exactly why soy is cut in your Detox phase—to prevent estrogen overload!

Cheeses and Yogurt

I know this might be a tough one, as cheese and yogurt are easy grab 'n' go proteins and they taste great. But both of these introduce two challenges. First, they are loaded with lactose (a sugar found in dairy). To efficiently digest lactose, your body produces an enzyme called lactase. When you don't have enough lactase, lactose can't be fully digested, causing bloating and gas (always fun!). The second challenge is that many people have a slight allergy to milk protein. The result can be excess mucus, which leads to head and chest congestion as well as inflammation. Now you might be thinking, *Where will I be getting my calcium?* Simple, add green leafy vegetables like spinach, kale, and collard greens and green vegetables like broccoli and asparagus to your plan. They are loaded with calcium and don't cause bloating.

► Exception

In step 2 of your Detox phase, Clean (your next step), I explain why it's important to have shakes as well as whole food in your meal plan. Two of the recommended shakes in your plan do contain some milk protein, Core Protein made by MYNT and Proto Whey made by Power

Crunch. Due to the way both of these shakes are made, you shouldn't experience any digestive challenges that you might encounter with whole-milk protein like cheese and yogurt. If you still experience digestive challenges, simply switch to egg-white protein or one of the recommended plant-based protein powders.

Refined Sugar

We often hear, "Avoid sugar." That statement doesn't make much sense since all carbohydrates (fruit, vegetables, and grains, with fiber being the exception) are metabolized into sugar. What you actually need to watch for is refined sugar, which is the added sugar that's found in candy, soda, most processed foods, and so on. Refined sugars include basically any sugar that's not naturally occurring in the food.

These types of sugars spike your blood sugar, which triggers fat storage and water retention.

Sugar-Free Sweeteners

Ever have gas when chewing sugar-free gum? It happens to most of us, and the culprit is the sugar-free sweetener in the gum. The most used sugar-free sweeteners include: aspartame, saccharine, sorbitol, xylitol, and sucralose. These are "fake" sugars that are formed with a double sugar molecule that your body can't digest. Since this molecule can't be digested, the result is gas and bloating. There is plenty of research that these once-touted calorie savers may actually be worse for your body than refined sugar is. The great news is, there is already a natural and healthy sweetener on the market called stevia, which can be digested by your body.

Salt

I remember watching my mom have some popcorn with her salt, seriously! And the next day she would share how puffy she felt. Adding salt to your food or eating processed food (which is loaded with salt) will cause massive bloating. Every milligram of sodium attracts water, causing your body to retain water. The more salt you eat, the more bloating you'll experience. In your Detox phase, the only salt you will have is the small natural amount in the clean foods you'll be eating. If you're a salt lover like my mom, no need to panic, in your Thrive phase, you can moderately add salt back into your plan. Your two best salt choices are sea salt and pink Himalayan salt, as both are natural and unprocessed and help minimize the bloating effects of regular table salt. Just remember to use them moderately.

Soda/Pop (Diet and Regular)

I know this isn't a shocker, as we're told by almost everyone to cut soda. There's a good reason to do this. All types of sodas are full of chemicals, carbonation (which causes gas in your intestines), and either refined sugar (regular soda) or sugar-free sweeteners (diet soda). What I've learned is people are attached to their soda, so I'm simply asking you to cut it for seven days. What you'll see is that seven days later, you won't crave soda anymore and you'll be less bloated. Double win!

Alcohol

Now you might be thinking, *I thought alcohol dehydrates me, so how can it bloat me?* Well you're right that it dehydrates you. When your body feels it doesn't have enough water, it shifts into water-retention mode to protect itself, primarily in terms of blood flow. In addition, alcohol disrupts your digestion by making your body metabolize the alcohol first (alcohol calories can't be used for energy) before your food is digested. Because of this digestion delay, there is a greater chance for your food to be stored as fat. Finally, alcohol disrupts your sleep cycles, and lower quality of sleep equals more stress, and that equals more bloating.

So just like soda, cut the alcohol for seven days. Then I'll show you how to moderately work alcohol back into your life a little at a time in your Thrive phase.

Coffee and Caffeinated Tea

Many of us love coffee and caffeinated tea—I know I do! They're cut from your Detox phase to help get your adrenal gland (your battery) cleaned up and to balance out your cortisol levels. The caffeine in coffee and tea triggers an over-release of adrenaline from your adrenal gland, which is then countered with a release of your stress hormone cortisol (too much cortisol in your body leads to unwanted belly fat). Most coffee and caffeinated tea drinkers have trained their bodies to rely on that caffeine rush—basically your body has become addicted to the caffeine. This causes you to use caffeine to mask some existing sleep deprivation and fatigue. Cutting caffeine will remove the fake energy mask and get your body back in balance.

You might be thinking, *What about decaffeinated coffee?* Well, coffee is very acidic, so even decaf coffee is something to cut in your Detox phase. However, the good news is that one to two cups a day of caffeine-free tea throughout your entire plan is just fine. Simply choose a good herbal tea, and bottoms up! And if you're a coffee and tea drinker who enjoys the caffeine, once detoxed, you'll be adding green tea in your Ignite phase to help burn fat, and coffee can be brought back in your Thrive phase.

> ## Exception

Caffeine withdrawal can cause throbbing headaches. When you cut caffeine, if you notice that your energy drops too low and you're experiencing headaches, you *can* add back one cup of caffeinated coffee or tea each day during the Detox phase. Drink that in the morning with your breakfast.

Grains and Calorie-Dense Vegetables

High-quality grains like quinoa, oatmeal, brown rice, and millet are amazing carbohydrates, as are calorie-dense vegetables like beans, sweet potatoes, and yams. They are all fiber-rich complex carbohydrates that slow down digestion and help keep blood sugar levels balanced. All these great benefits are exactly why you're cutting them for seven days. You heard me right—even though they are great carbs, they are also heavier and more calorie-dense carbohydrates, which can cause some additional water retention (since carbs attract water molecules just like sodium does). Your Detox phase is all about eating a diet as light and rich in nutrients and as easy to digest as possible. This is why your best carbohydrate choices in your Detox phase are fruits and low-calorie vegetables. No worries, though. In seven days you'll be loving your grains and calorie-dense vegetables once again.

Cut Your Exercise
(Only for Seven Days)

You must be thinking, *Mark, you're crazy. How can I lose weight by cutting my exercise?* Hold tight. I'm only talking no exercise for seven days. There are three great reasons to cut exercise during the Detox phase:

- Cleansing your body can be challenging—no need to put more stress on it with exercise. Remember, everything is about 1 percent. You'll be doing plenty of exercise in your Ignite phase, but the first step is to rock your Detox phase.

- As I shared earlier, most of us carry five to ten pounds of additional bloat that we will easily drop just by doing this seven-day detox, without exercise.

- No doubt exercise is how you maximize fat burning, but as important as exercise is, it can also cause water retention (inflammation) due to the temporary damage to your muscle tissue (that's the good soreness you feel after working out). Your goals in the Detox phase are to cleanse your body, flush your system, and remove as much inflammation as possible. This is best accomplished by not exercising in the seven-day Detox phase. And a good future note is, it's great to give your body a break from intense exercise every three months. It lets your body recover, heal, and come back stronger.

➤ **Exception**

You can do moderate exercise, like walking or a casual bike ride (fifteen to forty-five minutes' worth) during the Detox phase to keep your blood flowing and muscles moving. Stretching for ten minutes each night would also help optimize your detox.

➤ **Quick Detox Heads-Up**

If you've ever detoxed or cleansed before, you know it can be challenging the first few days. This seven-day detox is not nearly as aggressive as most. As I've shared, your blood sugar will be balanced the entire time and you're basically just eating super-clean food, cutting the junk, and giving your body a much needed oil change. With that being said, still be prepared for an energy drop in the first three days of your detox, and if you experience headaches, that's most likely from caffeine withdrawal. Simply follow the coffee and tea exception I shared earlier in this section. No worries, though—once your body cleans itself out, you'll be feeling like a champ.

Step 2: Clean

Where step 1 is all about cutting the bloating foods and having a seven-day vacation from exercise, step 2 is about simultaneously bringing in the right clean foods to replenish your body and balance your hormones. *Clean* means high quality, digestive friendly, and minimally processed—basically all-natural foods.

As I shared in chapter 2, you'll be eating in threes all day long, every three hours, with a balance of protein, fat, and carbs. Once you check out your meal plan, you'll see that you'll be eating whole, clean proteins (like chicken, egg whites, fish, and turkey) throughout the day. Since eating whole protein five times a day can tax your digestive system, it's important to add a clean shake a couple times a day to give your digestive system a bit of a break. This is because shakes are already in a liquid form so the digestive process has already started. This creates a perfect resting period between whole protein meals for your digestive tract. You'll be eating whole, clean proteins (as well as clean fats and carbs) for breakfast, lunch, and dinner, and clean shakes for your midmorning and midafternoon meals.

Besides the break that shakes provide your digestive system, they also are excellent for those grab 'n' go moments. I've honestly never met someone who's not busy. Each of us is classic at filling an already slammed schedule. This is why clean shakes are such a great element in your meal plan. They fill your eating gaps during the busiest times of the day, midmorning and midafternoon.

———————

There are two easy parts to your clean step:

- Add clean food.

- Turbocharge your detox with supplements.

➤ Important Note

Your plug-and-play Detox meal plan, portion sizes, exchange system, and detox-friendly recipes are presented at the end of this chapter.

Clean Proteins

Eat only these types of proteins in your Detox phase.

Lean Proteins

(high in protein, very low in fat)

- Bison (extra lean)

- Chicken

- Egg Whites

- Hemp (plant based, low in fat, ex. hemp powder)

- Lean fish (ex., bass, halibut, tilapia, tuna)

- Turkey

- Venison

Non-Lean Proteins

(high in protein and fat; do not add additional fat to a meal when eating these proteins)

- Hemp (plant based, regular fat content)

- Salmon

➤ Quick Detox Protein Tips

- Avoid any protein high in saturated fat in your Detox phase, like beef, pork, egg yolks, and lamb. Due to the saturated fat amounts and density levels, these proteins are harder for your body to digest. In addition, avoid shellfish during your Detox phase, like shrimp, crab, and lobster, as most shellfish are high in cholesterol. Both are added back in during your Ignite phase.

- If you prefer plant-based protein, simply choose plant-based powder proteins, hemp, and other plant-based options to ensure you are getting enough protein per meal. There are approved plant-based recipes for Detox, Ignite, and Thrive phases at the end of each phase chapter.

Protein Powder (Shakes)

Here's your protein powder litmus test to ensure you choose a quality shake:

- The powder needs at least 20 grams of protein per serving.

- There must be more protein than carbs and fat in the powder.

- The protein source needs to be one of these: whey (hydrolyzed, isolate, or concentrate), micellar casein, egg white, or plant based that does not contain soy protein. It can have trace amounts of soy in the form of soy lecithin, which has very little soy and is a binder in shakes.

- The powder needs to be gluten-free.

- The powder needs to be low in sugar and use a natural sweetener (like stevia).

There are a few good protein powders that use small amounts of sucralose (fake sugar). If sucralose causes you to experience digestive challenges, avoid it.

My top recommended types and brands of protein shakes are:

- Zen Fuze shakes, made by Jeunesse, with micellar casein and whey, all natural ingredients and flavored with stevia

- Power Crunch, Proto Whey made by BNRG with hydrolyzed whey

- Egg white protein powder—many quality brands and options

- Warrior Blend plant-based powder, made by Sunwarrior

- Vega One Nutritional Shake, plant-based powder, made by Vega

Clean Carbohydrates

Eat only fruits and nonstarchy vegetables for your carbohydrates in your Detox phase.

All Fruits

- Apples

- Bananas

- Berries

- Grapefruit

- Kiwi

- Mangos

- Melons

- Oranges

- And others

All Nonstarchy Vegetables

- Asparagus

- Broccoli

- Carrots

- Cucumber

- Green beans

- Peppers

- Squash

- Tomato

- And others

Clean Fats

Eat only these types of fats in the Detox phase.

- Avocado

- Chia seeds

- Flaxseeds or flax oil

- Natural nut butters (almond butter, peanut butter, etc.)

- Oils (coconut, macadamia, olive)

- Raw nuts (almonds, cashews, pecans, etc.)

Clean, Free Foods

The following foods are all natural, very low in calories, and salt-free.

All Herbs

- Basil

- Bay leaves

- Cilantro

- Dill

- Parsley

- Rosemary

- Sage

- Thyme

- And others

All Spices

- Cinnamon
- Garlic
- Ginger
- Nutmeg
- Peppercorns
- Saffron
- And others

Leafy Greens (Fresh Only)

- Collard greens
- Kale
- Lettuce (all types)
- Spinach
- And others

➤ **Cool Spice Tip**

Mrs. Dash makes tons of tasty salt-free herbs and spices to keep your food flavorful without the bloat. You can find the Mrs. Dash collection in almost any grocery store. I suggest trying a new spice medley each month to keep your meals robust and different. Food variety is huge in staying consistent with your plan and preventing the number-one culprit from sneaking in and derailing your momentum: the dreaded food boredom.

► ## Three Guidelines to Follow with Your Foods

✔ **All protein, carbohydrates, and fats need to be fresh or flash frozen.** Most flash frozen foods will feature a *Flash Frozen* label on their package and it means to freeze rapidly to prevent the formation of ice crystals. Do not eat canned or other packaged foods, as they are loaded in nitrates, salt, and preservatives. Also avoid all processed deli meats.

✔ **If possible, buy organic.** Organic food is more pure and clean. Organic fruits and vegetables are filled with many more antioxidants since they are pesticide-free. Organic eggs and lean meats are better fed and cared-for animals and fish, which creates a better quality protein.

✔ **Use hormone-free protein.** Hormone imbalances cause havoc in your body. The last thing you want is to get additional hormones from your food.

Cleansing Supplements

Part of detoxing your body is cleaning out two very important organs that directly affect your metabolism, your liver and kidneys. Look at your liver as your body's digestive gatekeeper. Basically, 99 percent of everything you put in your mouth has to go through your liver. Your liver decides what gets kept out, what needs to be inspected a bit more, and what's allowed to be distributed throughout your body. Look at your kidneys like a pasta strainer or filter. Similar to your liver, your kidneys keep some things in your body that you need and get rid of the other things you don't. There are four important things your kidneys do: make urine, control your body's chemical balances, remove wastes and excess fluid from your blood, and help control your blood pressure.

The other really important piece to turbocharging your detox is cleaning out your colon (large intestine). Even though cleaning out your colon is definitely not tons of fun or that pretty of an image, it's very important in optimizing your digestive system during your Detox phase and preparing your digestive tract to be revved up during your Ignite phase.

You will be effectively cleaning your liver, kidney, and colon just by following the three steps of your Detox phase—Cut, Clean, and Flush. The goal with taking additional natural supplements is to kick your detox into high gear and to turbocharge the cleansing of your liver, kidneys, and colon to maximize your detox results. Below are the four recommended supplements and a brief description of what they do.

▶ **Quick Note**

The recommended dosage and the time of day you should take each supplement are based on what research supports and on what I and our Venice Nutrition practices have seen work best for all who have experienced the plan. You will be able to get these recommended products at your local vitamin store, health facility, or online and there are specific high-quality brands of these products that I and our nutrition practices recommend and that can be found in the reference section at the back of this book.

> ## Very Important

If you have any medical challenges or are taking any type of medication, *always* check with your doctor before adding any supplementation.

Liver Detox Supplement

MILK THISTLE (SILYMARIN)

Milk thistle is a plant with seeds that contain a group of three compounds—silibinin, silidianin, and silicristin. These compounds are collectively known as silymarin. Silymarin has been used for more than two thousand years to treat gallbladder and liver disorders as well as help cleanse the liver.

Recommended daily dosage: 500 mg (100 mg of silybum marianum) once a day

Kidney Detox Supplement

CRANBERRY

Cranberries are a great kidney detoxifying food. They have been shown to help clean your kidneys in two ways:

1. Some of the chemicals in cranberries prevent bacteria from sticking to the cells that line the urinary tract, where they

can multiply. This greatly assists with keeping your urinary tract clean.

2. Cranberry contains significant amounts of salicylic acid. Salicylic acid helps reduce swelling, prevents blood clots, and can have antitumor effects.

Recommended daily dosage: 500 mg once a day

Colon/Intestine Detox Supplements

DANDELION ROOT AND DIGESTIVE ENZYMES

1. Dandelion root is an herb with diuretic properties that also assists in liver cleansing and is rich in fiber to help with digestion and proper intestinal health.

2. Digestive enzymes provide your body with the necessary enzymes (lactase, lipase, protease, amylase, cellulose) to assist in metabolizing food and strengthening your intestines.

Recommended daily dosage: Dandelion root—1500 mg once a day. Digestive Enzyme Blend—250–300 mg once a day

PSYLLIUM HUSK

A natural fiber that provides added bulk in your colon to improve regular bowel movements, psyllium husk will be used in the Detox phase and will be recommended for you as well during your Ignite and Thrive phases. If you currently have consistent bowel movements (at least once a day), you don't need to take this additional fiber in your Ignite and Thrive phases.

Recommended daily dosage: 5 g (capsule or powder form) twice a day

Step 3: Flush

It's a given that to detox, you need to be drinking water. Imagine cleaning a really dirty bowl or glass without any water. How would you get all the grime and dirt out? You wouldn't. The exact same thing applies to your body. Your body needs water consistently to flush out toxins, hydrate your skin, and maintain healthy blood volume, and your body needs it to lose weight. Your water is being taken to a new level these next seven days. Basically, the more you can drink (within the recommendations), the better. It's time to flush your system.

Here are your recommendations:

✔ **Females:** 2–4 liters per day (8–16 8-ounce glasses)

✔ **Males:** 3–5 liters per day (12–20 8-ounce glasses)

▶ **Two Quick Flush Tips**

- If you're currently not drinking water or have preexisting water retention problems, slowly increase your water consumption during your Detox, Ignite, and Thrive phases. This gradual increase will help your body adapt to its new hydration levels. Always remember, the goal is 1 percent improvements, so just focus on drinking a little more water each day.

- Steaming and sitting in a sauna are excellent ways to flush additional toxins during your Detox phase. Here's how to maximize a steam or sauna experience:

  1. Take a warm shower to open up your pores.

  2. Go in the steam or sauna for 5–10 minutes (until it feels too hot).

3. Immediately take a 1-minute cold shower or jump in a cold plunge pool (spas have these). This closes your pores.

4. Repeat the cycle of steam/sauna followed by cold shower or plunge pool one to two additional times. Each hot/cold cycle will help release more bloat and toxins from your body than if you just sit in the steam or sauna for the same period of time.

5. Make sure to drink plenty of water throughout this process, and if you feel light-headed or dizzy, immediately stop and remove yourself from the sauna, steam, or water. There is a caution, though: this method is only for those in good health and free of any cardiac concerns. As always, it is best to consult your physician when starting any new health regimen.

Your Plug-and-Play Detox Plan

The number-one request from clients is they want to keep things simple and basically just be guided on exactly what to do. I totally get that, and I also know that for parents, the need for simplicity is multiplied by ten, at least! Bottom line, we all need and want information quickly and easily because with the busy lives we live, it can be challenging to sort through the data. This is exactly why your Detox, Ignite, and Thrive plans are designed to be pure plug and play. In this chapter, as with your Ignite and Thrive chapters, the main steps from each chapter will be featured and your meal plan, food choices, portion sizes, and exchange system are all grouped together in a simple plug-and-play fashion. Basically, look, read, and do. It's that easy!

> ### ➤ Quick Family Note

As parents, the last thing we want is to make different meals for ourselves and then for our families. Your Detox, Ignite, and Thrive plans are 100 percent family friendly. The entire plan is centered on eating in threes and is high-quality whole food. Hunter has eaten this way since he stopped breastfeeding, and he follows the flexibility of the Thrive phase. The only things not for your kids are the cleansing, fat-burning, and digestive supplements, presented throughout the phases—those are designed just for adults.

Your plug-and-play plan for the Detox phase is on the following five pages.

PHASE 1

DETOX
LOSE YOUR BLOAT

GUIDELINES FOR YOUR DETOX PHASE

Important Note

Extend your Detox phase to 14 days (instead of 7) if one or more of these describes you:

- You have 50 lbs. or more to lose
- You drink alcoholic beverages 3+ times per week
- You are a smoker

Guidelines to Optimize Your Portion Sizes:

✓ Let go of the calorie mind-set. Simply follow the portion sizes and meal plan designed for your gender.

✓ You can measure your portion sizes by weight or with your hands (palm, fist, and thumb). Do whatever is easiest and most convenient.

✓ Make sure you're hungry (ready to eat but never starving) before each meal and satisfied (never full) after. If you're hungry before 3 hours, simply eat a balanced meal before the 3-hour mark.

✓ If you measure food with a scale, always measure it precooked since weight will be lost during cooking. If you measure portion sizes with your hands, always measure after it's cooked (only applies to cooked food).

Guidelines to Optimize Your Results:

✓ You will be eating in threes: eating every 3 hours with a balance of protein, fat, and carbs.

✓ Eat your first meal within an hour of waking and your last meal within an hour of bedtime.

✓ If you fall off your Ignite or Thrive plan for more than 3 days, you can reboot your plan by simply repeating this 7-day Detox phase.

✓ If you prefer a shake for breakfast, simply switch your breakfast and midmorning meals.

✓ Add a 6th meal if you're still hungry after dinner: have a shake or a meal with protein + carb + fat.

✓ **Supplements are optional. They are designed to turbocharge your results.** ◆

◆ Specific recommended brands of shakes and supplements can be found in the reference section.

PHASE 1 DETOX
LOSE YOUR BLOAT

WEEK 1 OF YOUR 8 WEEK RUN

1 CUT

CUT the foods and drinks that cause bloating.

Below is a list of foods and drinks that cause water retention:

- Gluten
  (found in most bread products)
- Soy
- Cheese & Yogurt
- Refined Sugar
- Sugar Sweeteners
  (besides stevia)
- Salt
- Grains
- Soda Pop (diet & regular)
- Alcohol [1]
- Caffeinated Coffee & Tea [2]

Also Cut Exercise [3]

1 Cut alcohol during Detox & Ignite phases.

2 If you experience headaches, you can have one cup of caffeinated coffee or tea in the morning. Decaffeinated herbal tea is fine throughout your Detox phase.

3 Exercise can cause inflammation. Your goals in Phase 1 Detox: clean your body, flush your system, and remove as much inflammation as possible. This is best accomplished by NOT exercising in the seven-day Detox phase (moderate exercises like walking 30–45 minutes at a time is fine).

2 CLEAN

Add the **CLEAN** foods & supplements to cleanse your body.

SAMPLE MEAL PLAN
see next page for suggested meal portions + foods

Breakfast	Protein + Carb + Fat (Ex.: Egg Whites + Berries + Almonds)
Midmorning	Protein Shake ◆ (see list on next page)
Lunch	Protein + Carb + Fat (Ex.: Chicken Breast + Green Beans + Avocado) (also take Cleansing Supplement with meal)
Midafternoon	Protein Shake ◆
Dinner	Protein + Carb + Fat (Ex.: Grilled Halibut + Asparagus + Olive Oil + Medium Bowl of Spinach or Lettuce)

3 FLUSH

FLUSH the toxins from your system with H_2O.

Water Recommendations

FEMALES

2–4 Liters / Day

8–16 Glasses (8 oz.)

MALES

3–5 Liters / Day

12–20 Glasses (8 oz.)

Drink water with each meal and between each meal.

Drink as much water as you can within the recommended guidelines.

If you're currently not drinking water or have preexisting water retention problems, slowly increase your water consumption during your Detox, Ignite, and Thrive phases. This gradual increase will help your body adapt to its new hydration.

Using a steam or sauna is an excellent way to help sweat out the toxins!

◆ **Specific recommended brands of shakes and supplements can be found in the reference section.**

PHASE 1 — DETOX
LOSE YOUR BLOAT

SPECIAL NOTE: Any protein, carb, or fat can be exchanged for a different protein, carb, or fat; just swap from the list.

PORTION EXCHANGE SYSTEM & RECOMMENDED FOODS

PROTEINS	CARBOHYDRATES	FATS	FREE FOODS
PORTION SIZES	**PORTION SIZES**	**PORTION SIZES**	**PORTION SIZES**
FEMALES — MALES	FEMALES — MALES	FEMALES — MALES	NO LIMITS
1 PALM — 1½–2 PALMS	1 FIST — 2 FISTS	1 THUMB — 1 BIG THUMB	
(3 OUNCES) — (5 OUNCES)	(3 OUNCES) — (5 OUNCES)		

CHOOSE 1 PER MEAL	**CHOOSE 1 PER MEAL**	**CHOOSE 1 PER MEAL**	**UNLIMITED**
✓Lean Proteins [1]	✓Fruits	✓Avocado	✓Herbs
• Bison *(extra lean)*	• Apples	✓Chia Seeds	• Basil
• Chicken	• Bananas	✓Flax Seeds	• Bay Leaves
• Egg Whites	• Berries	✓Natural Nut Butters	• Cilantro
• Hemp *(low in fat, ex. hemp powder)*	• Grapefruit	*(1 tbsp. - for females)* *(1½ tbsp. - for males)*	• Dill
• Lean Fish *(no shellfish) (ex. halibut, tilapia, tuna, etc.)*	• Mangos	✓Oils	• Parsley
• Turkey	• Oranges	*(½ tbsp. for females)* *(1 tbsp. for males)*	• Rosemary
• Venison	• etc.	• Olive	• Sage
✓Non-Lean Proteins *(do not choose additional fat w/ these proteins)*	✓Vegetables [3]	• Coconut	• Thyme
• Hemp *(regular fat content)*	• Bell Peppers	• Macadamia	• etc.
• Salmon	• Broccoli	✓Raw Nuts	✓Spices
✓Protein Powder *(shakes)* [2] ◆	• Carrots	*(½ oz. ~ small handful - for females)* *(1 oz. ~ medium handful - for males)*	• Cinnamon
• Whey & Micellar Casein: Zen Fuze Shake *(made by Jeunesse)*	• Cucumber		• Garlic
• Hydrolyzed Whey: Proto Whey	• Squash		• Ginger
• Plant Based: Vega One or Warrior Blend	• Tomato		• Nutmeg
• Egg White: Many Quality Brands	• etc.		• Peppercorns
			• Saffron
	3 Avoid calorie dense veggies like beans, corn, peas, potatoes during Detox phase.		• etc.
			✓Leafy Greens *(fresh only)*
1 Only fresh, no processed meats and no beef, pork, or lamb - can add back in Ignite phase.			• Collard Greens
			• Kale
2 Avoid ALL protein bars during Detox.			• Lettuce *(all types)*
			• Spinach
			✓Natural Sweetener
			• Stevia

◆ Specific recommended brands of shakes and supplements can be found in the reference section.

PHASE 1	DETOX LOSE YOUR BLOAT	SPECIAL NOTE: Repeat the meal plan below each day for the next **1 WEEK** (7 days).

SUGGESTED MEAL PLAN

Detox Meal Plan for Females

	1 PROTEIN	1 CARB	1 FAT	SUPPLEMENTS
	SERVING SIZE	SERVING SIZE	SERVING SIZE	SEE BELOW FOR SUPPLEMENT SERVING SIZE
	1 PALM (3 OUNCES)	**1 FIST** (3 OUNCES)	**1 THUMB**	
Breakfast	3 Egg Whites (or 3 oz. protein from list)	3 oz. Fruit or Vegetables	½ oz. raw nuts (a small handful) (or choose 1 serving of fat from list)	**Fiber** • Psyllium Husk: 5 g (~ 1 heaping tsp.)
Midmorning	1 Shake Serving ◆ (serving size is based on nutrient label; use only water for your desired consistency)			
Lunch	3 oz. Protein	3 oz. Fruit or Vegetables	1 oz. Avocado (or 1 serving of fat from list)	**Cleansing** ◆ (take with your meal) • Milk Thistle: 500 mg (100 mg Silybum Marianum) • Cranberry Extract: 500 mg • Dandelion Root: 1500 mg • Digestive Enzymes Blend • **OR can take** Zen Prime: 2 Tablets **to replace all above**
Midafternoon	1 Shake Serving ◆ (serving size is based on nutrient label; use only water for your desired consistency)			
Dinner	3 oz. Protein	3 oz. Fruit or Vegetables **FREE FOOD** Medium Bowl of Spinach or Lettuce	½ tbsp. Oil (use the oil for your salad) (or choose 1 serving of fat from list)	**Fiber** • Psyllium Husk: 5 g (~ 1 heaping tsp.)
Late night	Shake or Meal Consisting of Protein, Fat, & Carbs *meal optional - eat if hungry*			

Water Recommendations
2–4 Liters / Day
8–16 Glasses (8 oz.)

Drink water with each meal and between each meal.

◆ Specific recommended brands of shakes and supplements can be found in the reference section.

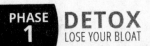

PHASE 1 · DETOX
LOSE YOUR BLOAT

SPECIAL NOTE:
Repeat the meal plan below each day for the next **1 WEEK** (7 days).

SUGGESTED MEAL PLAN

Detox Meal Plan for Males

	1 PROTEIN	1 CARB	1 FAT	SUPPLEMENTS
	SERVING SIZE	SERVING SIZE	SERVING SIZE	SEE BELOW FOR SUPPLEMENT SERVING SIZE
	1½–2 Palms (5 ounces)	**2 Fists** (5 ounces)	**1 Big Thumb**	
Breakfast	5 Egg Whites (or 5 oz. protein from list)	5 oz. Fruit or Vegetables	1 oz. raw nuts (a small handful) (or choose 1 serving of fat from list)	**Fiber** • Psyllium Husk: 5 g (~1 heaping tsp.)
Midmorning	1–2 Shake Servings (based on your level of hunger) ◆ (serving size is based on nutrient label; use only water for your desired consistency)			
Lunch	5 oz. Protein	5 oz. Fruit or Vegetables	2 oz. Avocado (or 1 serving of fat from list)	**Cleansing** ◆ (take with your meal) • Milk Thistle: 500 mg (100 mg Silybum Marianum) • Cranberry Extract: 500 mg • Dandelion Root: 1500 mg • Digestive Enzymes Blend • **OR can take** Zen Prime: 2 Tablets **to replace all above**
Midafternoon	1–2 Shake Servings (based on your level of hunger) ◆ (serving size is based on nutrient label; use only water for your desired consistency)			
Dinner	5 oz. Protein	5 oz. Fruit or Vegetables **FREE FOOD** Medium Bowl of Spinach or Lettuce	1 tbsp. Oil (use the oil for your salad) (or choose 1 serving of fat from list)	**Fiber** • Psyllium Husk: 5 g (~1 heaping tsp.)
Late night	Shake or Meal Consisting of Protein, Fat, & Carbs *meal optional - eat if hungry*			

Water Recommendations
3–5 Liters / Day
12–20 Glasses (8 oz.)

Drink water with each meal and between each meal.

◆ Specific recommended brands of shakes and supplements can be found in the reference section.

DETOX
Approved Recipes

The simplicity of your seven-day Detox meal plan is what makes it so easy and effective—you just repeat the same meal plan for seven straight days. For many people that is great, while others get bored after day one. Well, if you like a little more variety and wonder how that's possible with such a small food list, this section is made for you! Here are your Detox approved recipes, and you can eat them at any meal. For your convenience and time efficiency, each recipe will have one of these two labels (this applies to all recipes in this book):

- **Grab 'n' Go:** 10 minutes or less, for when you're in a time crunch

- **Gourmet Style:** 30 minutes or less and perfect for a nice dinner with your family and/or friends

> ## Important Recipe Notes for Your Detox, Ignite, and Thrive Phases

Venice Nutrition Head Chef Valerie Cogswell and I oversaw the recipes provided for all three phases. This collection is a mixture of recipes developed by Chef Valerie, Venice Health Professionals, and other 8 Week Runners just like you. All of us working together to create simple, tasty, and balanced recipes that make clean food taste great! Chef Valerie has also provided her top recipes for each phase—these recipes have two asterisks (**) by the recipe title.

The recipes for all three phases are presented in the order of breakfast, lunch, dinner, shakes, and plant based. In your Thrive phase, there are bonus dessert and side dish sections. The calories and macronutrient breakdowns (protein, carbohydrates, and fat) are listed based on serving size, and each recipe can be eaten anytime throughout the day. Follow the portion sizes presented in your plug-and-play meal plans, and remember to stay focused on eating in threes. Please note that because these recipes are a collection from various contributors, some recipes include ingredients measured in cups while other recipes include ingredients measured in ounces, depending on the individual contributor's preference and recipe style.

Each recipe features a balance section that either tells you the recipe itself provides the correct balance of macronutrients (protein, carbohydrates, and fat) or gives you the specific sides to eat along with the recipe to provide that balance. Easy to follow so there is no guessing!

Keep your meals balanced, and if it's time to eat and you're not hungry, simply cut your meal in half based on your portion sizes.

Breakfast

Spicy Fiesta Egg Scramble with Avocado and Cilantro**

Add some life to your eggs in only ten minutes with this simple, vibrant dish. Try chopping veggies in bulk for the week for quick grab 'n' go meals like this one.

Makes 1 serving

Serving size: 1 scramble
Calories per serving: 200
Protein per serving: 16 grams
Carbohydrates per serving: 18.5 grams
Fat per serving: 8 grams

   Fat-free cooking spray

   ½ cup chopped bell pepper (red, yellow, orange, green, or combo)

   ¼ cup chopped red onion

   **⅓ small jalapeño, finely chopped (or more depending on
      desired heat)**

   ½ cup grape tomatoes, sliced in half

   Cayenne pepper

   Black pepper

   4 egg whites

   1½ ounces avocado, chopped

   Fresh cilantro, chopped for garnish

   ½ orange (for garnish)

1. Heat a nonstick frying pan over medium-high heat. Coat pan with fat-free cooking spray.

2. Sauté bell peppers, onion, jalapeño, and half the tomatoes for 3 minutes. Season with desired amount of spices.

3. Push veggies to the side of the pan and add egg whites. Cook until scrambled, about 3 to 4 minutes.

4. Top eggs and veggies with remaining tomatoes, avocado, and plenty of fresh cilantro. Add a squeeze of fresh orange juice over the top.

What Is the Balance?

This recipe has a great balance of protein, carbohydrates, and fat.

Grab 'n' Go

Egg White Banana Pancake

Whip up a deliciously sweet, super-clean pancake with this fast and easy recipe!

Makes 1 serving

Serving size: 2 pancakes
Calories per serving: 188
Protein per serving: 11 grams
Carbohydrates per serving: 17 grams
Fat per serving: 7 grams

3 egg whites

1 tablespoon almond butter or your favorite nut butter

½ banana

Pinch of cinnamon (optional)

Fat-free cooking spray

1. Combine egg whites, nut butter, banana, and cinnamon in a blender until smooth.

2. Cook batter like you would pancakes, using fat-free cooking spray.

What Is the Balance?

This recipe has a great balance of protein, carbohydrates, and fat.

Grab 'n' Go

Chicken Salad with Kale, Pears, and Citrus Herb Vinaigrette**

Dress up your salad with a shot of sweet citrus and thyme dressing. Dark leafy greens, like kale, add powerful vitamins and minerals. We recommend that you cook chicken breast in bulk for easy grab 'n' go meals like this one all week long. You can also reserve leftover dressing for salads later in the week.

Makes 1 serving

Serving size: 1 salad
Calories per serving: 247
Protein per serving: 19.5 grams
Carbohydrates per serving: 23 grams
Fat per serving: 9 grams

FOR THE DRESSING

1 shallot, finely chopped

Juice from 1 small lemon

Juice from 1 large orange

3 sprigs thyme, leaves removed and chopped

2 tablespoons olive oil

Black pepper

⅓–½ packet stevia (depending on desired sweetness)

FOR THE SALAD

3 ounces cooked chicken breast, chopped or shredded

1 large handful kale (chopped very small) or your favorite greens

½ pear, thinly sliced

½ carrot, grated (optional)

1. Whisk together the first four ingredients for the salad dressing (shallots through thyme).

2. Slowly whisk in olive oil until a dressing forms.

3. Add freshly ground black pepper.

4. Taste and add as much stevia as desired.

5. Combine salad ingredients.

6. Pour salad dressing over salad ingredients.

What Is the Balance?

This recipe has a great balance of protein, carbohydrates, and fat.

Grab 'n' Go

Egg White Salad with Pesto

Plain old egg whites get a fun makeover with basil pesto. We recommend hard-boiling eggs in bulk for easy grab 'n' go meals like this one all week long. Use leftover pesto to dress up chicken, fish, or your favorite salad.

Makes 1 serving

Serving size: 1 salad
Calories per serving: 156
Protein per serving: 21 grams
Carbohydrates per serving: 5 grams
Fat per serving: 8 grams

FOR PESTO

1 bunch basil

4 tablespoons olive oil

1 tablespoon water

3 tablespoons pine nuts

4 large cloves garlic

Juice from 2 large lemons

FOR EGG SALAD

3 hard-boiled egg whites cut into bite-size pieces

1 ounce diced celery

1 ounce diced white onion

1 ounce diced tomato

1. Combine all pesto ingredients in a food processor and pulse until creamy.

2. Combine all egg salad ingredients in a small bowl.

3. Add 1½ tablespoons of pesto to egg salad and toss gently.

What Is the Balance?

To balance the meal, simply add a small side of fruit or vegetables. This will provide a great balance of protein, carbohydrates, and fat.

Dinner

Gourmet Style

Baked Fish in Foil with Tomato, Pineapple, and Cilantro**

This family-friendly recipe boasts simple ingredients, easy preparation, and easy cleanup with tons of bold flavor. Serve the fish straight out of the foil with all of its natural sauce in the Detox phase. In the Ignite and Thrive phases, you can serve it on top of brown jasmine rice.

Makes 4 servings

Serving size: 4 ounces fish
Calories per serving: 216
Protein per serving: 24 grams
Carbohydrates per serving: 11.5 grams
Fat per serving: 9 grams

1 pound any white fish

Freshly ground black pepper

1 tablespoon extra virgin olive oil

1 cup chopped pineapple

1 cup cherry or grape tomatoes, sliced lengthwise

½ cup chopped white onion

5 cloves garlic, smashed

Handful cilantro, roughly chopped

A few chives, chopped

Juice from ½ orange

Juice from ½ lime

Cilantro for garnish

1. Preheat oven to 350°F. Place one or two large pieces of tinfoil down in a baking pan and place fish on top—you want to form a large pocket for the fish to steam inside of the foil without any juices escaping.

2. Season fish with pepper and drizzle with extra virgin olive oil.

3. Add pineapple, tomatoes, onions, garlic, cilantro, and chives on top.

4. Squeeze orange and lime juice over the top.

5. Fold top of foil to make a pocket (making sure that the juice can't escape from the top or bottom of the pocket).

6. Bake for about 25 minutes, or until fish is cooked through. Top with plenty of fresh cilantro and serve the fish with the natural sauce that forms in the tinfoil pocket.

What Is the Balance?

This recipe has a great balance of protein, carbohydrates, and fat.

Gourmet Style

Lime-Mint Grilled Chicken with a Watermelon Avocado Salsa

This easy dish can be prepared ahead of time so dinner is a breeze. Make the marinade early in the day and marinate the chicken for at least 3 hours or overnight. You can prep the salsa ahead of time too. The result? A light, refreshing, and delicious meal that takes only minutes to put together.

Makes 5 servings

Serving size: 3¼ ounces chicken plus salsa
Calories per serving: 193
Protein per serving: 20 grams
Carbohydrates per serving: 12.5 grams
Fat per serving: 6.5 grams

FOR THE MARINADE

¼ cup fresh mint

2 tablespoons fresh parsley

1 jalapeño

Juice from 4 limes

1 clove garlic

Freshly ground pepper

1 pound chicken breast

FOR THE SALSA

5 ounces avocado, chopped

10 ounces watermelon, chopped

9 ounces seedless cucumber, chopped

2 tablespoons fresh mint, chopped

3 ounces red onion, chopped

1–2 jalapeños (depending on desired heat), chopped

Juice from 1 lime

1. Puree all the ingredients for the marinade in a food processor or blender. Pour over chicken and marinate for at least 3 hours.

2. Toss salsa ingredients in a small bowl and allow flavors to blend.

3. Grill marinated chicken for approximately 4–6 minutes per side, or until cooked through.

4. Top with fresh salsa.

What Is the Balance?

This recipe has a great balance of protein, carbohydrates, and fat.

Baked Lemon-Herb Salmon

This simple, heart-healthy dish requires very little preparation and is best served with a vegetable of your choice for a balanced meal. Leftovers can be used for a salad topping later in the week.

Makes 5 servings

Serving size: 4 ounces salmon
Calories per serving: 213
Protein per serving: 29 grams
Carbohydrates per serving: 0.5 grams
Fat per serving: 10 grams

Nonfat cooking spray

1 1½-pound salmon fillet

Freshly ground black pepper

10 fresh chives

4 thyme sprigs

4 oregano sprigs

4 rosemary sprigs

1 medium onion, sliced

½ lemon

Lemon slices for garnish

1. Preheat oven to 450°F.

2. Line shallow roasting pan with foil; coat with cooking spray.

3. Place fish on prepared pan and sprinkle with pepper.

4. Arrange chives, thyme, oregano, and rosemary horizontally across fish. Arrange onion slices on top of herbs.

5. Squeeze fresh lemon juice on top.

6. Cover with foil; seal. Bake 20–25 minutes, or until fish flakes easily when tested with a fork.

7. Serve warm or at room temperature with lemon slices for garnish.

What Is the Balance?

This dish is made of protein and fat. Please add a carbohydrate such as spinach or asparagus on the side for a complete meal.

Shakes

Grab 'n' Go

Piña Colada Smoothie

Fuel your body and burn fat with this easy tropical fruit smoothie.

Makes 1 serving

Serving size: 1 shake
Calories per serving: 218
Protein per serving: 21 grams
Carbohydrates per serving: 20 grams
Fat per serving: 7.5 grams

> **1 scoop Zen Fuze vanilla protein powder (or your favorite vanilla protein powder)**
>
> **1 teaspoon coconut oil**
>
> **½ ounce banana**
>
> **1 ounce pineapple**
>
> **Water**
>
> **Ice**

1. Combine all ingredients in a blender until smooth.

What Is the Balance?

This recipe has a great balance of protein, carbohydrates, and fat.

Grab 'n' Go

Mint Chocolate Smoothie

Got cravings? Indulge in a chocolate mint smoothie that is actually good for you.

Makes 1 serving

Serving size: 1 shake
Calories per serving: 150
Protein per serving: 21 grams
Carbohydrates per serving: 14 grams
Fat per serving: 3 grams

1 scoop Zen Fuze chocolate protein powder (or your favorite chocolate protein powder)

7–8 fresh mint leaves

1 drop peppermint extract (optional and can only be used in Ignite and Thrive phase)

Water

Ice

Organic chocolate shavings as garnish (optional and can only be used in Thrive phase)

1. Combine all ingredients in a blender until smooth.

2. Garnish with chocolate shavings, optional and only in Thrive Phase

What Is the Balance?

This recipe has a good balance of protein, carbohydrates, and fat. The carb and fat grams are a little low in this meal. If hungry, please feel free to add a little extra fruit and nuts on the side for a more filling meal.

Plant Based

Due to the high amount of carbohydrates found in most plant-based options, these plant-based recipes will be less balanced than the other recipes provided in this book. To boost your protein in these recipes, add a plant-based protein shot on the side. Some options for your protein shot are Vega One, Warrior Blend, or a low-fat hemp powder. Simply take a scoop of the protein powder, mix it in water, and drink it before or along with your meal. This will help balance out your meal.

Gourmet Style

World-Famous Magic Mushrooms

These protein-packed mushroom caps will have you seeing fungi in a whole new light. The rich, bold flavor of the caps along with a robust salad and some nuts on the side make a delicious meal.

Makes 4 servings

Serving size: 2 mushroom caps, 3 cups salad, approximately
    3 tablespoons nuts/seeds
Calories per serving: 287
Protein per serving: 18 grams
Carbohydrates per serving: 38 grams
Fat per serving: 11 grams

8 large portobello mushroom caps

6 cloves garlic, whole

Splash of red wine vinegar

Dried basil

8 cups baby spinach

2 cups cherry tomatoes, whole

2 cups sliced baby peppers

1 cup shredded carrots

1 cup shredded beets

¼ cup raw cashews

¼ cup raw, shelled pistachios

¼ cup raw pumpkin seeds

2 limes

1. Sauté the mushroom caps and whole garlic cloves with a splash of red wine vinegar and basil to taste in a saucepan on low heat until soft, about 10 minutes; plate.

2. Combine the spinach, tomatoes, and baby peppers into your favorite salad arrangement; place alongside the mushroom salad.

3. Place shredded carrots and beets on top of each salad.

4. Mix the cashews, pistachios, and pumpkin seeds together and serve on the side or add crunch to the salad by pouring them on top.

5. Cut each lime in half. Squeeze fresh lime over the salads right before serving.

What Is the Balance?

Add a plant-based protein shot from Vega One or Warrior Blend (or any brand that passes your protein powder litmus test explained in the Clean step of the Detox chapter and in the supplement reference section at the back of this book) or a low-fat hemp powder. Simply take a scoop of the plant-based protein powder, mix it in water, and drink before or along with your meal. This will provide a solid balance of protein, carbohydrates, and fat.

Garden Bowl Delight

This lightly cooked, low-fat veggie salad is served in an edible bowl and packed with nutrients.

Makes 4 servings

Serving size: 1 large cabbage leaf bowl, 2 cups (cooked) veggies
Calories per serving: 178
Protein per serving: 8 grams
Carbohydrates per serving: 24 grams
Fat per serving: 5 grams

2 cups chopped broccoli

2 cups chopped tomatoes

2 cups chopped butternut squash

2 cups chopped peppers

6 cloves garlic, whole

4 cups baby spinach

No-salt grill seasoning

2 tablespoons olive oil

1 large head red cabbage

1. Add all veggies except the cabbage to a saucepan.

2. Season to taste with no-salt grill seasoning.

3. Add olive oil and cook over medium heat until soft (the veggies should retain most of their bright color).

4. Separate the cabbage head into individual leaves.

5. Place one leaf inside another to make a two-layer bowl.

6. Pour cooked veggies into cabbage leaf bowls and serve.

What Is the Balance?

Add a plant-based protein shot from Vega One or Warrior Blend (or any brand that passes your protein powder litmus test explained in the Clean step of the Detox chapter and in the supplement reference section at the back of this book) or a low-fat hemp powder. Simply take a scoop of the plant-based protein powder, mix it in water, and drink before or along with your meal. This will provide a solid balance of protein, carbohydrates, and fat.

There you have it, a safe and simple seven-day Detox plan that cleans out your system and sets your body up to win. It's time your inflated weight became a thing of the past and your bloat disappeared forever. Dive into your plug-and-play plan, rock this week, and next week you roll right into Phase 2: Ignite, where you're going to turn your body into a fat-burning machine and melt your belly with your next three steps—Burn, Sculpt, and Restore!

4

IGNITE:
Melt Your Belly

Weeks 2–4: Burn, Sculpt, Restore

On the surface most of us have been here before. Extra bloat dropped, scale quickly going in the right direction, inches shrinking, looking leaner, clothes fitting more loosely, and overall feeling better. All the signs of progress . . . but there is a difference this time. The difference is that you didn't lose your bloat through some miracle diet or magic pill; you legitimately lost your bloat and your inflated weight. You did it the right way, no shortcuts, no starvation, no carb depletion—you did it by eating in threes. You cut processed and bloating foods, added in clean and high-quality foods, and increased your water intake to flush out your toxins. Plus you cleansed three crucial parts of your digestive system: your liver (your body's clearing house) your kidneys (your body's filter), and your colon (your body's garbage truck). In essence you gave your body a complete oil change and created the perfect environment for your body to win these next seven weeks as you enter your Ignite phase.

Tracey Regan also experienced these positive benefits as she entered her Ignite phase. She was super motivated, yet hesitant, wondering if this was too good to be true. As an athlete, mom, and wife, she had been at this place before. One solid week under her belt left her feeling good but she also questioned if she could keep it up. You see, in the past, Tracey never understood how her body was using the food she was eating, and she had never lived following a realistic plan that could work for her and her family. When she felt bloated and the scale was on the high side, she simply went to what she knew—cutting calories and increasing her exercise, basically starving herself and overexercising. She would drop the weight, burn some fat, and then a month or two later, everything she lost would be regained. That repeated experience made her hesitant now.

But as Tracey dove into her Ignite phase, she realized this wasn't anything she had done before. She was actually eating the foods she liked, exercising moderately, and as each week passed, her plan evolved into a way of life. Then after eight weeks, Tracey experienced something new: real results that stuck. Tracey lost twenty-four pounds, ten inches, and three sizes during her 8 Week Run and has dropped another ten pounds, two inches, and two sizes in her Thrive phase. And now check out her guns!

Just like Tracey did, you're going to light your furnace, ignite your metabolism, and turn your body into a fat-burning machine!

Tracey Regan

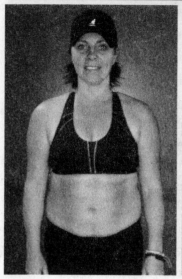
before

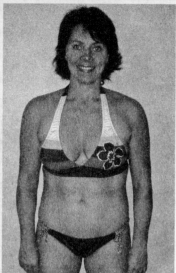
after 8 weeks

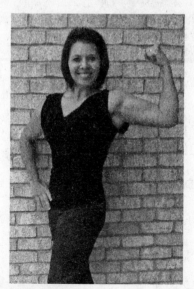
beyond 8 weeks

Quick 8 Week Run Weight-Loss Tip

Your Ignite phase will keep pounds and inches dropping and your belly fat melting. The average weight lost in the 8 Week Run (Detox, Ignite, and Thrive phases combined) is twenty-five to thirty pounds. Of course some people drop more than thirty pounds and some drop less. Once again, it all depends on the speed of your metabolism and your starting weight. In addition, even though you'll be burning lots of fat, it's important to understand that your body just can't continue to drop at the same pace as it did in your Detox phase. Remember, that was your inflated weight. In your Ignite phase, the average weight loss is about three pounds a week, which is a safe, realistic, and great weekly number. Stay the course, implement the strategies, and follow your plan. You're taking your body to the next level! Always remember, 1 percent at a time.

Three Steps to Ignite: Burn, Sculpt, Restore

Just like your Detox phase, your Ignite phase is as easy as 1, 2, 3:

- **Step 1:** Burn

- **Step 2:** Sculpt

- **Step 3:** Restore

You burn your fat by adding more food—a sixth meal and a metabolism booster—you sculpt your body with cardio and strength training, and you restore your digestive system with probiotics.

Important Note

In your Ignite phase, you'll be following the same principles as you did in your Detox phase. You're still cutting your bloating foods, eating clean foods, and drinking your H_2O. Each phase is designed to build off the previous phase, which helps create a consistent overall meal and exercise structure. In addition, each phase provides new adjustments to keep your results flowing and to evolve your plan into a way of life. To always maintain the theme of simplicity, your plug-and-play Ignite meal plan is presented at the end of this chapter, followed by your Ignite recipes.

Step 1: Burn

In your Detox phase, you focused on five meals a day and eating only simple and easily digestible carbohydrates (fruits and vegetables). That works great for seven days and does exactly what it's designed to do—detox your body and help you lose your bloat. But as the novelty of the plan wears off, you need to be ahead of the curve and prevent the statement we've all made: "Oh no, not another egg white or piece of chicken" (or whatever food you need a break from).

Bottom line, boredom with what you are eating leads to burnout, and burnout leads to quitting the plan, so variety matters. In addition, by eating in threes, your body is consistently releasing stored fat, and every pound of stored fat has 3,500 calories. The leaner you get and the less fat you have, the fewer stored fat calories your body has for energy. This causes you to get hungrier sooner between meals. Your body can only digest a certain amount of food per meal, so you're always better off adding another meal to your day than eating bigger meals. Your body is also a refuel-as-it-goes machine, meaning it needs to be fed consistently to stay in balance, release stored fat, and protect muscle.

For these reasons you'll be adding some additional proteins, carbs, and fats to your Ignite phase meal plan as well as an additional meal (if you're hungry) in your day. Plus you'll be replacing your cleansing supplements with some metabolism boosters to help turbocharge your fat burning. Let's start with the new foods you'll be eating.

New Ignite Phase Foods

Additional Lean Proteins

You pretty much had complete freedom with lean proteins in your Detox phase, with one big exception, shellfish. It's time to bring back your favorite shrimp, lobster, crab, and clam dishes. All shellfish is back on plan, so if it's one of your favorite proteins, go have some fun!

- Shrimp

- Lobster

- Crab

- Clams

- And others

Additional Non-Lean Proteins

In your Detox phase salmon and hemp were your only non-lean protein options. It's time to expand that list and add some additional variety. Non-lean protein options, like beef, are excellent sources of protein, but they have a good amount of saturated fat and are harder for your body to digest. An important thing to remember is that non-lean proteins have fat in them, which means they provide both your protein and your fat for a meal. So when you eat one of these proteins, don't add any additional fat to your meal.

- Beef (filet mignon and ground 99% lean)

- Egg yolk

- Lamb

- Pork tenderloin

Grains/Calorie-Dense Carbohydrates

These complex carbs are great to keep you satisfied longer between meals. Just be aware that since they take longer to digest and are more dense, they can cause bloating. Only add these carbs in one to two of your meals per day, and if you feel they bloat you, focus primarily on fruits and low-calorie vegetables as your carb choices instead. Remember, your portion sizes are the same in this phase, so be cautious with these carbs—small amounts can be packed with calories.

- Beans
- Brown rice
- Millet
- Oatmeal
- Potatoes (preferably sweet potatoes)
- Quinoa
- Yams

Fats

Most fats are heavily processed, so fat options are still a bit limited in this phase. The good news is, there is one to add, and it's one of Hunter's favorite foods.

- Olives—watch the sodium, though, and choose the most natural and freshest ones you can find.

Condiments

You already have some excellent free foods to make your food taste great and some creative recipes to keep things interesting. Here are two more free foods to spice things up a bit.

- Extract (almond, vanilla, etc.)
- Vinegar (balsamic, apple cider, red wine, etc.)—just beware of added sugar and sodium

Protein Bars and Ready-to-Drink (RTD) Shakes

These are much more processed than protein powder (shakes) and are really just for emergencies. At the most, have only one of these per day. I'll give you a litmus test for choosing a protein bar or RTD (ready to drink). It's similar to the guidelines I shared in the Detox chapter when choosing a protein powder. I also recommend a few of my favorite bars and RTDs on the market.

Protein bar and RTD shake litmus test:

- The protein in the bar or RTD needs to be within a five gram range of the total carbs. For example, if the food label shows twenty grams of carbohydrates, you can eat a bar that has anywhere between fifteen and twenty-five grams of protein. Staying within this five gram range ensures the bar or RTD will be correctly balanced. If the bar has more than five grams more carbs than protein, do not eat it; it will most likely spike your blood sugar.

- The protein source needs to be one of these—whey (hydrolyzed, isolate, or concentrate), micellar casein, egg white, or plant based that does not contain soy protein. It can have trace amounts of soy in the form of soy lecithin, which has very little soy and is a binder in most protein products.

- The bar or RTD needs to be gluten-free.

- The bar needs to be low in sugar, preferably high in fiber, and use a natural sweetener (like stevia). Most RTDs use small amounts of sucralose (fake sugar). If sucralose causes you to experience digestive challenges, avoid it.

A few recommended brands of protein bars and RTDs that pass this litmus test are:

- **Bars:** Power Crunch (preferably gluten-free options), Quest (choose flavors that pass litmus test), Rise Protein

- **RTDs:** Power Crunch (all flavors), Muscle Milk (all flavors), Premier Protein (all flavors)

Unsweetened Almond Milk and Coconut Water for Shakes

In your Detox phase, you used only water with your shakes—that's always your best choice for optimal results. I also know it can be fun and tasty to mix your shakes up with a couple low-calorie, clean, and healthy liquids. To keep the liquid excitement flowing, feel free to occasionally add up to a half cup of unsweetened almond milk or coconut water (the more natural, the better) to your shake. Just make the necessary adjustments with your other carbs to account for the additional calories. For example, if you normally add fresh berries to your shake, just add fewer berries to help offset the calories and carbs from the almond milk or coconut water.

▶ **Cool Recipe Tip**

If you really want to keep it clean, check out the Homemade Almond Milk recipe on page 136.

Add a Sixth Meal

The best sign that your metabolism is on fire is a feeling of hunger (ready to eat, not starving) every three hours and satisfaction after each meal (not full). As I shared, the leaner you get and the more consistent you are with your mealtimes, the more your body will trust that food is coming and will burn energy (your stored fat) that much faster. It's a foreign concept to most of us that we actually have to eat more to permanently lose weight, but hey, that's physiology and the science of how our body works!

Think of when your kids are growing or are more active—they need more fuel and eat more meals. It's the same reason you need to eat more the leaner you get and the more active you become. The leaner you are, the less stored fat you have, which means the additional calories your body needs must come from your meals.

► **Quick Reminder Note**

If you're currently eating five meals and don't have an appetite or any sense of hunger, simply cut your meals in half (maintaining the balance of protein, fat, and carbs) and still eat every three hours. Your appetite will awaken. Once you begin to get hungry every three hours (your body's way of telling you that it's time to eat) shift back to your recommended portion sizes.

Adding your sixth meal is optional, based on your appetite. Just continue to listen to your body, and remember, it is better to eat an additional meal than it is to eat bigger meals.

Turbocharge Your Fat Burning with Metabolism Boosters

Every day we hear about "incredible" fat burners on the market and how there is a new product that melts fat away regardless of your food and exercise. That hype is what I can't stand about the supplement industry. The most important thing to remember is that your number-one supplement is real food, period.

Supplements are designed to do exactly what their name says—supplement an already solid plan based on real food—and when used correctly, they help turbocharge your results. I've been using metabolism boosters since 1993. Basically, a quality metabolism booster is a product or combination of products that gently and gradually increases the speed of your metabolism without blowing your fuse. Most of us have experienced the blown fuse (I know I have!). It's the feeling after you've taken an appetite suppressant, fat burner, or aggressive energy drink and you feel like someone shot you with a vial of adrenaline. You start bouncing off the walls, getting jittery and shaky, shortly followed by an epic energy crash. This type of stimulus creates havoc on your adrenal gland (your body's battery) and causes hormone imbalances with adrenaline (your energy hormone) and cortisol (your stress hormone).

Just like how eating in threes keeps your blood sugar hormone levels balanced, it's important when using a metabolism booster to keep your energy and stress hormone levels balanced as well. These recommended metabolism boosters will prevent you from having those vicious energy swings that can derail your progress, and they'll still provide the fat-burning turbocharge you want.

► **Quick Note**

The recommended dosage and the time of day you should take each supplement are based on what research supports and what I and our Venice Nutrition practices have seen work best for all who have experienced the plan.

You will be able to get these recommended products at your local vitamin store, health facility, or online, and there are specific high-quality brands of these products that I and our nutrition practices recommend and that can be found in the reference section at the back of this book.

► **Very Important**

If you have any medical challenges or are taking any type of medication, always check with your doctor before adding supplementation.

Green Tea Extract

For centuries the Far East has known the power of green tea extract for weight loss, blood sugar balance, and antioxidant protection. There are four main benefits to green tea extract that will assist you in burning fat:

- It's rich in antioxidants. Antioxidants neutralize free radicals and protect healthy cells. Fewer free radicals keep your cells strong and your metabolism working better.

- It has EGCG (Epigallocatechin gallate), which helps with fat oxidation (breaking down fat and using it for energy).

- The polyphenols found in green tea extract help balance blood sugar by reducing the amount of amylase that's in your body. Amylase is the enzyme that converts starch to sugar, so less amylase slows down the rate of starch being converted to sugar, helping regulate your blood sugar levels.

- It enhances thermogenesis (production of heat) in your body, which increases fat metabolization (fat burning). What's even better is it does this without increasing your heart rate, unlike many other thermogenic supplements, which means no jitters—very nice!

Recommended daily dosage: 250 mg (50 percent caffeine) twice a day, 30 minutes before your meal

Chromium Polynicotinate

Chromium is an essential mineral that approximately 80 percent of the population may be deficient in. Chromium polynicotinate is chromium combined with vitamin B$_3$, also known as niacin. The combination of the two has been shown to help insulin (one of your blood sugar hormones) better utilize glucose and shuttle it more efficiently to your cells. This helps balance your blood sugar, and more stable blood sugar equals the release of more stored fat. Something we all want.

Recommended daily dosage: 200 mcg twice a day, 30 minutes before your meal with the green tea extract

Step 2: Sculpt

We each have the vision of the toned body we want—maybe it's defined arms, lean stomach, tight glutes, and shaped legs. Sculpting your body is getting that look you want, whatever it may be. As you eat in threes, your body releases your stored fat, and that fat gets burned up in your muscle. To optimize your fat burning and truly sculpt your body, it's all about working out smarter and more efficiently.

Too many times people hit a plateau they can't break through, and it's due to their lack of exercise diversity. We fall into a rut of doing the same types of workouts that originally got us results. The problem is, your body is an ever-adapting machine and within weeks it can adapt to an exercise routine. Once it adapts, that workout shifts away from sculpting your body and toward simply maintaining your results. The way you prevent an exercise rut is to correctly diversify your workouts with the three types of exercise.

> ## Quick and Important Exercise Note

In this book there are two exercise sections. This section provides you with a basic structure to optimize your workouts and ensure you are doing all three types of exercise. But I also get that as a parent, even though many times we know what to do, we can't find the time to do it. That's what chapter 7, "It Looks Like a Gym to Me," is all about, finding creative and realistic ways to squeeze your exercise in throughout your day. So look at this section as your exercise plan for when you have the time to follow a solid routine, and at chapter 7 as your free-flowing exercise plan for when time is tight and you need to bring the gym to you!

Three Types of Exercise

- **Fat-burning cardio:** This includes any moderate exercise like walking, stair-climbing, cycling, jogging, or swimming—

basically when you have a steady heart rate and you're not winded. Fat-burning cardio activates your body's red muscle, which is about 50 percent of your skeletal muscle, meaning the muscles you voluntarily control. This means that if you can move it—like when you lift your arm, scratch your back, or walk up stairs—you are using skeletal muscle.

- **High-intensity cardio:** This is better known as interval training, which is characterized by bursts of speed (high heart rate) followed by recovery periods (lower heart rate). Some examples are sprinting, jumping rope, spinning, running stairs, boxing, or most ball sports (like singles tennis, racquetball, basketball, and soccer). Basically, anything that has bursts of speed followed by moments of recovery. High-intensity cardio activates your body's white muscle, which is approximately the other 50 percent of your skeletal muscle.

- **Strength training:** This is any type of exercise that overloads your muscles and causes them to become stronger. A few examples are weight training, Pilates, yoga, kettlebells, CrossFit, and exercises like push-ups, pull-ups, and squats. Always remember, more muscle equals a faster metabolism, so strength training is great for men and women, and it's been shown to help improve bone density as well.

The opposite page has a quick snapshot of how to structure your workouts to get all three types of exercise in, recruit both your red and white muscle, maximize your fat burning, and increase your lean body mass (muscle). Simply adjust the recommended days to match your schedule.

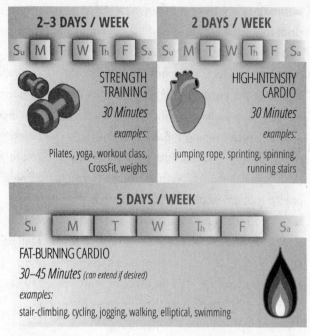

2–3 DAYS / WEEK

Su M T W Th F Sa

STRENGTH TRAINING
30 Minutes

examples:

Pilates, yoga, workout class, CrossFit, weights

2 DAYS / WEEK

Su M T W Th F Sa

HIGH-INTENSITY CARDIO
30 Minutes

examples:

jumping rope, sprinting, spinning, running stairs

5 DAYS / WEEK

Su M T W Th F Sa

FAT-BURNING CARDIO
30–45 Minutes (can extend if desired)

examples:

stair-climbing, cycling, jogging, walking, elliptical, swimming

NOTES:

Perform all strength training & high-intensity cardio **before** fat-burning cardio.

Sprinting or a sport like singles tennis, racquetball, basketball, etc. is the ideal high-intensity cardio. *For fun, cool, and creative ways to make exercise work as a parent, dive into chapter 7 of this book.*

► Quick and Important Exercise Tips

If you weren't exercising before you started your 8 Week Run, remember 1 percent improvements. Just start doing fat-burning cardio, and as you build consistency, start adding in some high-intensity cardio and strength training.

Always do your strength training and high-intensity cardio before your fat-burning cardio. It takes your body approximately twenty minutes to shift from burning primarily sugar to fat (first twenty minutes is 60 percent sugar, 40 percent fat, and then at the twenty-minute mark it shifts to 60 percent fat, 40 percent sugar, and the percentages continue to move more to fat burning for energy as exercise time increases). High-intensity cardio and strength training mostly burn sugar, so by doing your high intensity and strength training first, you deplete your body's sugar stores. Then as you shift into fat-burning cardio, you immediately tap in to your stored fat for fuel. This little adjustment will optimize your body's fuel pathways and maximize your results. Consider fast-paced sports with quick bursts of speed like singles tennis, racquetball, soccer, or basketball as high-intensity cardio.

The exercise graphic is just an example of how to diversify your exercise. If you already have a set exercise plan, keep rocking it. Just make sure it involves the three types of exercise—fat-burning, high intensity, and strength training. If you have never done strength training or haven't had instruction, I strongly suggest you initially work with a trainer, take a group class, or watch a video. It's impossible to achieve results if you're injured, and doing strength training incorrectly is a surefire way for that to happen.

Step 3: Restore

Your metabolism is only as strong as your digestive system, meaning regardless of how clean you eat, if your digestive system isn't working correctly, you can't metabolize your food and your results will suffer. This is why your Detox phase was so important. It cleaned your system and got your body to work optimally again. Now it's time to keep it healthy and strong. That's what your Restore step is all about.

Naturally, with eating clean, exercising efficiently, and staying hydrated, your body is working well. Now we want to turbocharge your results with some additional digestive, fiber, and omega-3 supplements to maximize your body's functionality. Here are the three recommended supplements for your Restore step:

PROBIOTICS

During digestion your body requires live bacteria to help metabolize food and move it through your gastrointestinal tract (stomach and intestines). You naturally have this bacteria, but many people lack the necessary amounts to efficiently digest their food. Add the additional stressors of life (especially for us parents!) that negatively affect your intestinal tract, and many of us need all the digestive help we can get. Enter probiotics, which are live bacteria strains that replace or add to the bacteria in your intestinal tract.

You have a few options when it comes to probiotics. You basically have three choices: one strain of bacteria, multiple strains of bacteria, or over-the-counter pharmaceutical probiotics. Here's an explanation of each:

- **One strain of bacteria:** An example is acidophilus, a bacteria that's typically found in dairy products and assists with digestion. Many people get this probiotic as a supplement from their local health food store. Just follow the suggested dosages on the bottle.

- **Multiple strains of bacteria:** Whereas acidophilus is an example of one strain, there are probiotic supplements that have multiple strains of bacteria to provide a full spectrum. Look for anything that has over 1 billion live cultures.

- **Pharmaceutical probiotic:** I always prefer natural probiotics, but in some cases, pharmaceutical probiotics are necessary based on an individual's digestive system. These are designed to help people with digestive challenges like irritable bowel syndrome, Crohn's disease, and colitis. I've worked with thousands of clients with these challenges, and probiotics definitely help.

➤ **Quick Probiotic Note**

For the brands of probiotics I recommend, please refer to the reference section in the back of this book. My personal preference is the multiple strain probiotics because they're natural and have a full variety of strains. This provides excellent assistance for your digestive tract.

OMEGA-3

Most likely, if you're not eating salmon or flaxseed every day, you're deficient in omega-3s. The strong nails and glowing skin we all want, along with lower blood pressure and cholesterol, and of course reduced joint pain and inflammation and better digestion, can all be attributed to getting enough omega-3 fatty acid in your meals. Essential fat means your body can't make it, but it needs it to optimally function, so you can either get it through your food or from supplements. Since most of us don't eat salmon daily (if you do, great job!), we need to supplement with omega-3s. Here are three easy ways to supplement:

1. Take a fish oil or flax gel cap (use a pharmaceutical grade).

2. Take flaxseed oil (but adjust your food balance for the 14 grams of fat in each tablespoon).

3. Use fresh flax, chia, or hemp seeds in your meals.

Recommended daily dosage: 3,000 mg per day

> ### Quick Omega-3 Note

For the brands of omega-3s I recommend, please refer to the reference section in the back of this book.

PSYLLIUM HUSK

You used psyllium husk in your Detox phase to provide fiber to help clean out your colon. Many people continue to use this fiber to maintain regular bowel movements (at least once per day). Being regular is extremely important to maximizing fat burning and maintaining a healthy digestive system. If you have a challenge with constipation, I strongly suggest continuing the use of this fiber supplement. If your bowel movements are now regular, then adding the fiber supplement is optional.

Recommended daily dosage: 5 g twice a day

Your Plug-and-Play Ignite Plan

Your plug-and-play plan for the Ignite phase is on the following five pages.

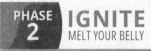

PHASE 2 IGNITE
MELT YOUR BELLY

GUIDELINES FOR YOUR IGNITE PHASE

Important Note

In your Ignite phase, you will be following the same principles as in your Detox phase, only your plan will be expanded to turn your metabolism into a fat-burning machine.

Guidelines to Optimize Your Portion Sizes (same as Detox phase):

✓ Let go of the calorie mind-set. Simply follow the portion sizes and meal plan designed for your gender.

✓ You can measure your portion sizes by weight or with your hands (palm, fist, and thumb). Do whatever is easiest and most convenient.

✓ Make sure you're hungry (ready to eat but never starving) before each meal and satisfied (never full) after. If you're hungry before 3 hours, simply eat a balanced meal before the 3-hour mark.

✓ If you measure food with a scale, always measure it precooked since weight will be lost during cooking. If you measure portion sizes with your hands, always measure after it's cooked (only applies to cooked food).

Guidelines to Optimize Your Results:

✓ New meal guidelines for Ignite phase:

⇨ If you fall off plan for more than 3 days, you can reboot your plan by simply repeating your 7-day Detox phase.

⇨ Add a sixth meal to attack stored fat (this meal is optional, only eat if hungry).

⇨ Add complex carbs to help keep you more satisfied.

⇨ Add additional protein, fat, and carb options to prevent boredom.

⇨ Add metabolism boosters to maximize fat burning.

⇨ You can have 1 protein bar or ready-to-drink shake at max per day (just for emergency in Ignite phase).

✓ Keep eating in threes and follow the mealtime and water guidelines presented in this phase (Ignite).

✓ **Supplements are optional. They are designed to turbocharge your results.** ◆

◆ Specific recommended brands of shakes, bars, & supplements can be found in the reference section.

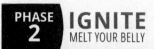

PHASE 2

IGNITE
MELT YOUR BELLY

WEEKS 2–4 OF YOUR 8 WEEK RUN

1 BURN

BURN your belly fat by adding more food, complex carbs, and metabolism boosters:

- Add a sixth meal to keep your body fueled and attack stored fat, especially your trouble areas.

- Add complex carbs like brown rice, quinoa, and sweet potatoes to a maximum of 2 of your meals per day to help keep you more satisfied. (Complex carbs can cause water retention, so only add daily if they do not cause bloating.)

- Add metabolism boosters to ignite your body's furnace and maximize fat burning.

- Repeat your Ignite Phase weeks 5–8 if your goal is to still lose weight and maximize fat burning.

2 SCULPT

SCULPT your body by activating your engine with cardio and strength training:

Sculpting is all about activating all your muscle and working out smarter, not harder.

Here is how to maximize your exercise: [1, 2]

2 DAYS / WEEK
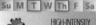
Su **M** T **W** **Th** F Sa

HIGH-INTENSITY CARDIO

30 Minutes

examples:
jumping rope, sprinting, spinning, running stairs

2–3 DAYS / WEEK
Su M T **W** **Th** **F** Sa

STRENGTH TRAINING

30 Minutes

examples:
Pilates, yoga, workout class, CrossFit, weights

5 DAYS / WEEK

Su **M** **T** **W** **Th** **F** Sa

FAT-BURNING CARDIO

30–45 Minutes
(can extend if desired)
examples:
stair-climbing, cycling, jogging, walking, elliptical, swimming

1 Perform all strength training and high-intensity cardio before fat-burning cardio.

2 Sprinting or a sport like singles tennis, racquetball, basketball, etc., is the ideal high-intensity cardio. *For fun, cool, and creative ways to make exercise work as a parent, dive into chapter 7 of this book.*

3 RESTORE

RESTORE your digestive system with probiotics:

Your Detox phase cleansed your body, and now it's time to Restore your digestive tract. Probiotics are live bacteria that help restore your digestive system and help in allowing your intestines to function optimally.

SAMPLE MEAL PLAN
see next page for suggested meal portions + foods

Breakfast	Protein + Carb + Fat (Ex.: Egg Whites + Oatmeal + Almonds) (with Essential Fats and Fiber Supplements) ◆
Midmorning	Protein Shake (with Fat Burning and Digestive Supplements from list) ◆ ◇
Lunch	Protein + Carb + Fat (Ex.: Salmon + Brown Rice + Asparagus)
Midafternoon	Protein Shake (with Fat Burning and Digestive Supplements from list) ◆ ◇
Dinner	Protein + Carb + Fat (Ex.: Steak + Broccoli + Spinach w/ Balsamic Vinegar) (with Fiber Supplements) ◆
Late night	Protein Shake OR Complete Meal *(this meal is optional, eat if hungry)*

PHASE 2

IGNITE
MELT YOUR BELLY

SPECIAL NOTE:
The same portion sizes and food exchange system guidelines in the Detox phase apply to the Ignite phase.

PORTION EXCHANGE SYSTEM & RECOMMENDED FOODS

★ New to Ignite phase

PROTEINS	CARBOHYDRATES	FATS	FREE FOODS
PORTION SIZES	**PORTION SIZES**	**PORTION SIZES**	**PORTION SIZES**

FEMALES   MALES
1 Palm   1½–2 Palms
(3 ounces)   (5 ounces)

FEMALES   MALES
1 Fist   2 Fists
(3 ounces)   (5 ounces)

FEMALES   MALES
1 Thumb   1 Big Thumb

NO LIMITS

CHOOSE 1 PER MEAL	CHOOSE 1 PER MEAL	CHOOSE 1 PER MEAL	UNLIMITED

PROTEINS — CHOOSE 1 PER MEAL

✓Lean Proteins
- Bison *(extra lean)*
- Chicken
- Egg Whites
- Hemp *(low in fat, ex. hemp powder)*
- Lean Fish *(shellfish is now okay) (ex. tuna halibut, tilapia, etc.)*
- Turkey
- Venison

✓Non-Lean Proteins *(do not choose addl. fat w/ these proteins)*
- ★ Beef *(filet mignon)*
- ★ Beef *(ground 99% lean)*
- ★ Eggs, Whole
- ★ Fish *(non-lean) (ex. salmon)*
- Hemp *(regular fat content)*
- Lamb
- ★ Pork Tenderloin

✓Protein Powder *(shakes)* ◆
- Whey & Micellar Casein: Zen Fuze Shake *(made by Jeunesse)*
- Hydrolyzed Whey: Proto Whey
- Plant Based: Vega One or Warrior Blend
- Egg White: Many Quality Brands

CARBOHYDRATES — CHOOSE 1 PER MEAL

✓Fruits
- Apples
- Bananas
- Berries
- Grapefruit
- Mangos
- Oranges
- etc.

✓Vegetables
- Bell Peppers
- Broccoli
- Carrots
- Cucumber
- Squash
- Tomato
- etc.

✓Grains/Calorie-Dense Veggies [1] *(choose gluten-free when relevant)*
- ★ Beans *(choose fresh/dried) (ex, black, kidney, garbanzo, etc.)*
- ★ Brown Rice
- ★ Millet
- ★ Oatmeal
- ★ Potatoes *(sweet potatoes are best)*
- ★ Quinoa
- ★ Yams

1 For grains/calorie-dense veggies, use hand sizes rather than weight.

FATS — CHOOSE 1 PER MEAL

✓Avocado
✓Chia Seeds
✓Flax seeds
✓Natural Nut Butters *(1 tbsp. for females) (1½ tbsp. for males)*
✓Oils *(½ tbsp. for females) (1 tbsp. for males)*
- Coconut
- Macadamia
- Olive
- ★ Olives [2]
✓Raw Nuts *(½ oz. – small handful - for females) (1 oz. – medium handful - for males)*

2 For olives, use hand sizes rather than weight.

FREE FOODS — UNLIMITED

✓Herbs
- Basil
- Bay Leaves
- Cilantro
- Dill
- Parsley
- Rosemary
- Sage
- Thyme
- etc.

✓Spices
- Cinnamon
- Garlic
- Ginger
- Nutmeg
- Peppercorns
- Saffron
- etc.

✓Leafy Greens *(fresh only)*
- Collard Greens
- Kale
- Lettuce *(all types)*
- Spinach

✓Natural Sweetener
- Stevia

✓Condiments
- ★ Extracts *(almond, vanilla, etc.)*
- ★ Vinegars *(balsamic, red wine, etc.)*

◆ Specific recommended brands of shakes, bars, & supplements can be found in the reference section.

PHASE
2

IGNITE
MELT YOUR BELLY

SPECIAL NOTE:
Repeat the meal plan below each day for the next **3 WEEKS**.

SUGGESTED MEAL PLAN

Ignite Meal Plan for Females

	1 PROTEIN	1 CARB	1 FAT	SUPPLEMENTS
	SERVING SIZE	SERVING SIZE	SERVING SIZE	SEE BELOW FOR SUPPLEMENT SERVING SIZE
	1 PALM (3 OUNCES)	**1 FIST** (3 OUNCES)	**1 THUMB**	
Breakfast	3 Egg Whites (or 3 oz. protein from list)	1 Fist Oatmeal (1 small bowl) (or 3 oz. carbs from list)	½ oz. or Small Handful of Nuts (or choose 1 serving of Fat from list)	**Essential Fats ◆** • Omega-3 Fatty Acids: 3000 mg **Fiber** • Psyllium Husk: 5 g (~ 1 heaping tsp.) ‡
Midmorning	1 Shake Serving ◆ (serving size is based on nutrient label; for best results, use water. If needed can add up to ½ cup of unsweetened almond milk or coconut water)			**Digestive ◆** • Pro-Biotic: 1 capsule **OR** 1 Zen Fuze Shake **Fat Burning ◆ ◇** • Green Tea Extract (50% Caffeine): 250 mg • Chromium Polynicotinate: 250 mg • **OR** Zen Shape: 2 Capsules **can replace both plus enhanced fat burning**
Lunch	3 oz. protein	3 oz. carbs	1 serving fat	
Midafternoon	1 Shake Serving ◆ (serving size is based on nutrient label; for best results, use water. If needed can add up to ½ cup of unsweetened almond milk or coconut water)			**Digestive ◆** • Pro-Biotic: 1 capsule **OR** 1 Zen Fuze Shake **Fat Burning ◆ ◇** • Green Tea Extract (50% Caffeine): 250 mg • Chromium Polynicotinate: 250 mg • **OR** Zen Shape: 2 Capsules **can replace both plus enhanced fat burning**
Dinner	3 oz. protein	3 oz. carbs	1 serving fat	**Fiber** • Psyllium Husk: 5 g (~ 1 heaping tsp.) ‡
Late night	Shake or Meal Consisting of Protein, Fat, & Carbs *meal optional - eat if hungry*			

‡ Fiber Supplements are optional if having daily bowel movements. ◇ Take fat burning supplements 30 min. before a meal.

Water Recommendations
2–4 Liters / Day
8–16 Glasses (8 oz.)

Drink water with each meal and between each meal.

◆ Specific recommended brands of shakes, bars, & supplements can be found in the reference section.

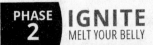

PHASE 2 **IGNITE** MELT YOUR BELLY

> **SPECIAL NOTE:**
> Repeat the meal plan below each day for the next **3 WEEKS**.

SUGGESTED MEAL PLAN

Ignite Meal Plan for Males

	1 PROTEIN	1 CARB	1 FAT	SUPPLEMENTS
	SERVING SIZE	SERVING SIZE	SERVING SIZE	SEE BELOW FOR SUPPLEMENT SERVING SIZE
	1½–2 PALM (5 ounces)	2 FISTS (5 ounces)	1 BIG THUMB	
Breakfast	5 Egg Whites (or 5 oz. protein from list)	2 Fists Oatmeal (1 medium bowl) (or 5 oz. carbs from list)	1 oz. or Medium Handful of Nuts (or choose 1 serving of Fat from list)	**Essential Fats** ✦ • Omega-3 Fatty Acids: 3000 mg **Fiber** • Psyllium Husk: 5 g (~ 1 heaping tsp.) ‡
Midmorning	1–2 Shake Servings (based on your level of hunger) ✦ (serving size is based on nutrient label; for best results, use water. If needed can add up to ½ cup of unsweetened almond milk or coconut water)			**Digestive** ✦ • Pro-Biotic: 1 capsule **OR** 1 Zen Fuze Shake **Fat Burning** ✦ ◇ • Green Tea Extract (50% Caffeine): 250 mg • Chromium Polynicotinate: 250 mg • **OR** Zen Shape: 2 Capsules **can replace both plus enhanced fat burning**
Lunch	5 oz. protein	5 oz.carbs	1 serving fat	
Midafternoon	1–2 Shake Servings (based on your level of hunger) ✦ (serving size is based on nutrient label; for best results, use water. If needed can add up to ½ cup of unsweetened almond milk or coconut water)			**Digestive** ✦ • Pro-Biotic: 1 capsule **OR** 1 Zen Fuze Shake **Fat Burning** ✦ ◇ • Green Tea Extract (50% Caffeine): 250 mg • Chromium Polynicotinate: 250 mg • **OR** Zen Shape: 2 Capsules **can replace both plus enhanced fat burning**
Dinner	5 oz. protein	5 oz. carbs	1 serving fat	**Fiber** • Psyllium Husk: 5 g (~ 1 heaping tsp.) ‡
Late night	Shake or Meal Consisting of Protein, Fat, & Carbs *meal optional - eat if hungry*			

‡ Fiber Supplements are optional if having daily bowel movements.   ◇ Take fat burning supplements 30 min. before a meal.

Water Recommendations
3–5 Liters / Day
12–20 Glasses (8 oz.)

Drink water with each meal and between each meal.

✦ Specific recommended brands of shakes, bars, & supplements can be found in the reference section.

IGNITE
Approved Recipes

Here are your Ignite approved recipes, and as with your Detox recipes, you can eat them at any meal. You can also use your Detox approved recipes because they work great in this phase too! Just like your Detox recipes, each recipe will be labeled:

- **Grab 'n' Go:** 10 minutes or less, for when you're in a time crunch

- **Gourmet Style:** 30 minutes or less and perfect for a nice dinner with your family and/or friends

▶ **Some Quick Recipe Reminders**

Venice Nutrition Head Chef Valerie Cogswell and I oversaw these recipes. This collection is a mixture of recipes developed by Chef Valerie, Venice Health Professionals, and other 8 Week Runners just like you. Chef Valerie has also provided her top recipes for each phase—these recipes have two asterisks (**) by the recipe title.

The recipes are presented in the order of breakfast, lunch, dinner, shakes, and plant based. The calories and macronutrient breakdowns (protein, carbohydrates, and fat) are listed based on serving size, and each recipe can be eaten anytime throughout the day. Follow the portion sizes presented in your plug-and-play meal plans, and remember to stay focused on eating in threes.

Each recipe features a balance section that either tells you the recipe itself provides the correct balance of macronutrients (protein, carbohydrates, and fat) or gives you the specific sides to eat along with the recipe to provide that balance. Easy to follow so there is no guessing!

➤ Quick Note

If you're not bored with your Detox foods or recipes and are loving the way you're feeling, you definitely do not need to add any of these new foods or recipes right now. They are completely optional. You can keep following your current plan, but you'll probably still need to add a sixth meal—but only if you're hungry.

Breakfast

Gourmet Style

Banana Quinoa Pancakes with Berry Syrup**

Move over, pancakes! These Ignite phase–friendly Banana Quinoa Pancakes are comfort food at its finest. Packed full of high-quality whole foods and fragrant spices, this nutritious breakfast will satisfy your sweet tooth while keeping your blood sugar in check. Make quinoa in bulk for the week and store it in the fridge so you can quickly use it in recipes like this one. Because of the density of the quinoa, these cakes cook best low and slow in a high-quality, nonstick pan. These pancakes are delicious with or without the syrup and can be stored in the fridge in an airtight container for 3–4 days.

Makes 4 servings

Serving size: 2 pancakes (4″ each) plus approximately ¼ cup berry syrup
Calories per serving: 166
Protein per serving: 5.5 grams
Carbohydrates per serving: 23 grams
Fat per serving: 5.5 grams

FOR THE PANCAKES

1½ small, very ripe bananas

1 extra-large whole egg

2 extra-large egg whites

¾ cup cooked quinoa

1 tablespoon unsweetened almond milk

2 teaspoons unrefined coconut oil

1½ teaspoons pure vanilla extract

½ teaspoon baking powder

¼ heaping teaspoon cinnamon

3 good dashes of nutmeg

Fat-free cooking spray

FOR THE SYRUP

1½ cups frozen mixed berries (all natural, no sugar added)

½ tablespoon unrefined coconut oil

Few drops pure vanilla extract

½–1 packet stevia (depending on desired sweetness)

1. Puree all the pancake ingredients in a blender for 4 minutes.

2. In the meantime, heat a large, nonstick frying pan over medium heat for the quinoa cakes. Coat with fat-free cooking spray.

3. For the syrup, heat a separate small frying pan over low heat and add all ingredients except the stevia. Stir occasionally.

4. Once large frying pan is hot, add ¼ cup of pancake mix per cake (make 4 at a time) and cook for approximately 4–5 minutes for the first side, lowering the heat if necessary. The key is to cook low and slow! Once the pancake edges get firm, gently flip and cook for another

3–4 minutes, lowering the heat if necessary. Remove cooked pancakes and keep warm.

5. Right before serving, sweeten syrup with stevia.

6. Serve pancakes with berry syrup.

What Is the Balance?

This recipe has a great balance of carbohydrates and fat plus some protein. We recommend that you add additional lean protein on the side such as egg whites or a protein shake made of protein powder and water.

Veggies and Eggs in a Sweet Potato Muffin

These make very tasty muffins for breakfast, brunch, or any meal.

Makes 4 servings

Serving size: 3 muffins
Calories per serving: 182
Protein per serving: 12 grams
Carbohydrates per serving: 14 grams
Fat per serving: 8 grams

6 ounces shredded sweet potatoes

2 ounces shredded carrots (matchstick carrots work best)

1 tablespoon olive oil

1 tablespoon minced garlic (divided)

½ tablespoon fresh oregano

1 tablespoon fresh basil

Fat-free cooking spray

4 ounces of favorite veggies (such as broccoli, onions, and
    red pepper), chopped

Ground cumin to taste

Ground paprika to taste

12 ounces egg whites

3 eggs

1. Preheat oven to 400°F.

2. Mix shredded sweet potatoes, carrots, olive oil, half of the garlic, and the oregano and basil together.

3. Spray muffin tins generously.

4. Pour sweet potato mixture evenly into muffin tins, and press it down and on the sides, forming the mixture into "cups."

5. Bake until edges are brown, approximately 20 minutes.

6. While sweet potatoes are baking, spray a pan with fat-free cooking spray and sauté veggies of your choice with the remaining garlic, and the cumin and paprika.

7. Once sweet potato muffins are crispy around the edges, scoop even amounts of sautéed veggies into each cup.

8. Mix egg whites and eggs together, and pour equal amounts over veggies in each cup.

9. Bake for an additional 15 minutes.

What Is the Balance?

This recipe has a great balance of protein, carbohydrates, and fat.

Protein Power Oatmeal**

If you're short on time in the morning and in need of a fast breakfast, Protein Power Oatmeal is the perfect choice. Warm, creamy oats are combined with chocolate or vanilla protein powder and natural nut butter for a quick and tasty meal. For a change of pace, swap in nuts, peanut butter, or ground flaxseeds for the almond butter.

Makes 1 serving

Serving size: 1 bowl
Calories per serving: 270
Protein per serving: 25 grams
Carbohydrates per serving: 25 grams
Fat per serving: 8 grams

¾ ounce instant oatmeal, dry, unsweetened

1–2 scoops Zen Fuze vanilla or chocolate protein powder (or your favorite vanilla or chocolate protein powder; serving size depends on label; focus on 25 grams of protein)

½ tablespoon natural almond butter or natural peanut butter

1. Stir oats and water (for correct amount of water, see oatmeal package) in a bowl, and microwave on high according to package directions.

2. Very slowly, stir in desired amount of protein powder a little at a time until the mixture is smooth and creamy. Quick note: Because protein powders vary in sweetness, you may choose to only use half of your recommended

protein powder in your oatmeal. If so, please mix your remaining protein powder with water and drink on the side to ensure you are getting your recommended intake of protein.

3. Add natural almond butter or peanut butter and mix well.

What Is the Balance?

This recipe has a great balance of protein, carbohydrates, and fat.

Lunch

Gourmet Style

Lettuce-Wrapped Turkey Burger on Sweet Potato "Bun"

These lettuce-wrapped burgers are an easy, healthy version of a family favorite. They can even be made ahead of time and reheated.

Makes 5 servings

Serving size: 1 burger with "bun" and toppings
Calories per serving: 229
Protein per serving: 19 grams
Carbohydrates per serving: 23 grams
Fat per serving: 6 grams

FOR THE BURGERS

1 pound ground turkey (99 percent lean)

Mrs. Dash salt-free seasoning

13 ounces cooked sweet potatoes

Fat-free cooking spray

FOR THE TOPPINGS

Leaf lettuce

5 tablespoons homemade or natural, sugar-free salsa

5 ounces avocado, chopped

Onion slices (optional)

Tomato slices (optional)

1. Mix turkey and salt-free seasoning until combined.

2. Shape into 5 patties and grill on medium heat until cooked throughout, about 7–10 minutes or until no longer pink.

3. In the meantime, mash sweet potatoes with same seasoning and shape into 5 patties (they will be sticky). Sauté potato patties in a pan coated with fat-free cooking spray until lightly browned on both sides.

4. Place 1–2 leaves of lettuce on a plate. Top with the sweet potato "bun."

5. Add the turkey burger, salsa, avocado, and desired toppings.

6. Wrap lettuce around burger, pick up, and enjoy!

What Is the Balance?

This recipe has a great balance of protein, carbohydrates, and fat.

Grab 'n' Go

Warm Chicken and Shrimp Quinoa Salad with Dried Cranberries

This easy salad is both warm and substantial. Plus it has a fun sweet and spicy kick. Prepare chicken and shrimp in bulk for the week for easy grab 'n' go meals like this one.

Makes 1 serving

Serving size: 1 salad
Calories per serving: 256
Protein per serving: 22 grams
Carbohydrates per serving: 25 grams
Fat per serving: 6 grams

1 cup kale

Garlic powder

Cayenne pepper (optional)

⅓ cup cooked quinoa

1 tablespoon dried cranberries

¼ ounce sunflower seeds

2 ounces chicken breast, cooked

1 ounce shrimp, cooked

1. In a nonstick pan, sauté the kale until soft. Season with desired amount of garlic powder and cayenne pepper.

2. Add the quinoa, dried cranberries, and sunflower seeds and sauté for a minute or two or until the sunflower seeds are lightly toasted.

3. Add in the chicken and shrimp and sauté until warm.

What Is the Balance?

This recipe has a great balance of protein, carbohydrates, and fat.

Gourmet Style

Tuna with Quinoa, Red Peppers, and Basil

This is an ideal family meal, or you can portion out single servings. To make your own roasted red peppers, lightly brush red bell peppers with olive oil and grill or sauté until softened.

Makes 4 servings

Serving size: 1 plate
Calories per serving: 254
Protein per serving: 24 grams
Carbohydrates per serving: 20 grams
Fat per serving: 10 grams

FOR THE QUINOA

1 cup cooked quinoa, cooled

⅓ cup roasted red peppers

¾ cup diced scallions

FOR THE TUNA

4 cans tuna in water, drained well

Juice from 2 lemons

Zest from 1 lemon

¼ cup fresh basil

1 small clove garlic, minced

½ teaspoon ground pepper

2 tablespoons olive oil

1 teaspoon Mrs. Dash Onion and Herb

1 teaspoon Mrs. Dash Garlic and Herb

1. Combine ingredients for the quinoa.

2. In a separate bowl, combine ingredients for the tuna.

3. Mix contents from both bowls together and toss well.

4. Divide onto 4 plates.

What Is the Balance?

This recipe has a great balance of protein, carbohydrates, and fat.

Grab 'n' Go

Chicken Nachos over Homemade Sweet Potato Chips

This lean take on nachos takes only minutes to make if you have sweet potato chips prepared ahead of time for the week. Simply cut sweet potatoes in thin, even slices, coat lightly with fat-free cooking spray, season with Mrs. Dash seasoning of your choice, and bake at 450°F until crispy, about 20–30 minutes. Just keep an eye on the potatoes while they cook, as they tend to burn.

Makes 1 serving

Serving size: 1 plate
Calories per serving: 216
Protein per serving: 19.5 grams
Carbohydrates per serving: 18.5 grams
Fat per serving: 6 grams

3 ounces cooked chicken breast, shredded

Favorite Mrs. Dash seasoning

Large handful homemade sweet potato chips (recipe above)

1 ounce chopped tomatoes

½ ounce sugar-free salsa

1 ounce avocado, chopped

1. In a small bowl, toss chicken with desired amount of Mrs. Dash seasoning. Heat in microwave for 30 seconds.

2. Arrange sweet potato chips on a plate.

3. Place seasoned, shredded chicken on top. Add tomatoes, salsa, and chopped avocado. Add a sprinkle of Mrs. Dash seasoning on top if desired.

4. Optional: Heat entire plate in the microwave for about 45 seconds to warm it up.

What Is the Balance?

This recipe has a great balance of protein, carbohydrates, and fat.

Dinner

Gourmet Style

Cilantro-Rubbed Pork Tenderloin with Citrus Sauce**

"The other white meat" becomes something amazing when rubbed in garlic and cilantro and then smothered in a citrus sauce. Serve sliced pork and sauce over brown jasmine rice or regular brown rice. We recommend that you cook brown rice in bulk for the week to pair with easy meals like this one.

Makes 4–5 servings

Serving size: 4 ounces pork plus citrus sauce (*nutrition information does not include brown rice*)
Calories per serving: 238
Protein per serving: 24 grams
Carbohydrates per serving: 10 grams
Fat per serving: 9 grams

FOR THE PORK RUB

Small handful fresh cilantro, chopped

1 clove garlic, finely minced

Pinch of red pepper flakes

½ tablespoon extra virgin olive oil

1–1½ pounds pork tenderloin, brought to room temperature

Fat-free cooking spray

FOR THE CITRUS SAUCE

1 tablespoon extra virgin olive oil

1 shallot, finely chopped

2 cups real orange juice (We used 100 percent fresh-squeezed, all-
natural bottled juice.)

Small handful fresh cilantro, including stems

2 sprigs of fresh thyme, including stems

2 cloves garlic, peeled and left whole but smashed

Pinch of red pepper flakes

1. Preheat oven to 350°F.

2. Mix ingredients for pork rub in a small bowl and rub on all sides of pork tenderloin.

3. Heat a large frying pan over medium-high heat. Once hot, spray generously with fat-free cooking spray. Let pan heat up for another moment.

4. Add pork to pan and sear to a light golden-brown crust on all sides.

5. Place seared pork on a sheet pan covered in foil, and bake in oven for 18–25 minutes, or until cooked through (cooking time depends on the size of the pork). Let pork rest for at least 5 minutes before slicing.

6. While pork is in the oven, start on the sauce. In the same pan used to sear the pork, add olive oil and sauté shallots over medium-low heat for 2 minutes.

7. Add orange juice.

8. Scrape up brown bits on the bottom of the pan.

9. Add fresh cilantro, thyme, garlic, and red pepper flakes.

10. Reduce heat slightly and reduce sauce by half, stirring occasionally.

11. Once reduced, use a fork to remove garlic, thyme, and cilantro from the sauce and discard. Add any juices from the pork right into the sauce.

12. Serve pork with brown rice and sauce. Garnish with fresh orange slices and plenty of fresh cilantro.

What Is the Balance?

This recipe alone has a great balance of protein and fat. It is slightly low in carbohydrates. When you add a small amount of brown rice (females ¼ cup cooked, males ½ cup cooked) or a veggie on the side, the carbohydrates will be just right.

Gourmet Style

Fillet Lettuce Wraps with Grilled Pineapple Salsa

Lean beef is rubbed with pungent spices, grilled to perfection, and served in a lettuce wrap with smoky pineapple salsa in this family-style dish.

Makes 5 servings

Serving size: 1 wrap plus salsa
Calories per serving: 206
Protein per serving: 25 grams
Fat per serving: 8 grams
Carbohydrates per serving: 12 grams

FOR THE WRAPS

1 tablespoon cumin

1 tablespoon coriander

1 tablespoon garlic powder

½ tablespoon paprika

½ tablespoon chili powder (no salt added)

1 teaspoon cayenne pepper (plus extra for pineapple)

1 pound lean beef tenderloins

Lettuce leaves (Boston Bibb works great or choose your favorite

lettuce)

FOR THE SALSA

6 ounces fresh pineapple, cored and sliced in rings

Cayenne pepper (optional)

4 ounces vine tomatoes, chopped

2 ounces red onion, chopped

3 ounces sweet peppers, chopped

1 jalapeño, chopped

1 tablespoon fresh mint, chopped

½ cup fresh lime juice

1. Combine spices for the wraps in a bowl and rub on fillet. Grill to desired doneness.

2. While steak is on the grill, prepare pineapple rings for the salsa. If desired, sprinkle pineapple rings with cayenne pepper for added heat and grill on both sides.

3. Add grilled pineapple, tomatoes, onions, peppers, jalapeños, mint, and lime juice to a large bowl and stir to combine.

4. Slice the steak, put it in the lettuce leaves, and top with pineapple salsa.

What Is the Balance?

This recipe has a great balance of protein, carbohydrates, and fat.

Gourmet Style

Grilled Halibut with Avocado Béarnaise Sauce and Quinoa

We all love béarnaise sauce, but the two main ingredients are egg yolks and butter. Now we can enjoy this take on béarnaise without the guilt by using heart-healthy avocado! Prepare quinoa according to package directions in bulk for the week to have on hand for quick meals like this one. You can marinate the fish earlier and then grill before serving for more intense flavor.

Makes 5 servings

Serving size: 2½ ounces fish plus sauce and quinoa
Calories per serving: 197
Protein per serving: 20 grams
Carbohydrates per serving: 16 grams
Fat per serving: 6 grams

FOR THE FISH MARINADE

1 tablespoon fresh chives

1 tablespoon fresh dill

1 stalk fresh lemongrass, grated

Juice from ½ orange

Juice from 1 lemon

1 clove garlic

2 6-ounce halibut fillets

FOR THE AVOCADO BÉARNAISE SAUCE

Fat-free cooking spray

1 shallot, chopped

1 clove garlic, chopped

Juice from ½ lemon

1 teaspoon white wine vinegar

2½ ounces avocado

1 tablespoon fresh tarragon

FOR THE QUINOA

1 cup cooked quinoa

1. Blend all marinade ingredients in a food processor and pour over fish.

2. Grill fish on low until flaky, about 4 minutes per side. Do not overcook.

3. While fish is cooking, make the béarnaise sauce. Coat a pan with fat-free cooking spray and sauté shallots and garlic for about 5–6 minutes, or until soft. Start with shallots and add garlic for the last 1–2 minutes. Garlic tends to overcook before shallots are to desired doneness if put in together.

4. In food processor, puree shallot mixture, lemon juice, vinegar, avocado, and tarragon until creamy. You may need to add a touch of water to thin the sauce out.

5. Serve fish and sauce over quinoa.

What Is the Balance?

This recipe has a great balance of protein, carbohydrates, and fat.

Bonus

Gourmet Style

Homemade Almond Milk

Making your own almond milk is easier than you think! This version is scented with real vanilla bean and is lower in sodium than store-bought versions. Try using a milk nut bag—a reusable, nylon drawstring bag (find online). A cheesecloth will work too.

Makes 8 servings

Serving size: ½ cup
Calories per serving: 40
Protein per serving: 2 grams
Carbohydrates per serving: 3 grams
Fat per serving: 2.5 grams

   1 cup raw almonds

   Water (for soaking almonds overnight)

   3½ cups additional water

   1 whole vanilla bean, cut into quarters

   1 date

   Sprinkle of cinnamon

1. Add almonds to a bowl and cover with water. Soak overnight.

2. Drain and rinse almonds.

3. Put almonds in a blender with 3½ cups water, vanilla bean, and date. Blend for 1 minute.

4. Strain really well using a nut milk bag (or cheesecloth).

5. Pour strained almond milk back into the blender with a sprinkle of cinnamon and blend one more time for 30 seconds.

What Is the Balance?

Almond milk makes for a creamy alternative to dairy milk and can be used to add a new twist to a shake or to put the finishing touches on a balanced meal.

Shakes

Grab 'n' Go

Peaches and Cream Smoothie

This creamy, decadent smoothie will fill you up while keeping your waistline in check.

Makes 1 serving

Serving size: 1 shake
Calories per serving: 249
Protein per serving: 23 grams
Carbohydrates per serving: 25 grams
Fat per serving: 8 grams

    1 scoop Zen Fuze vanilla protein powder (or your favorite vanilla
        protein powder)
    ½ cup unsweetened almond milk
    1½ ounces frozen peaches
    Dash of cinnamon
    ½ cup water
    Ice

1. Combine all ingredients in a blender until smooth.

What Is the Balance?

This recipe has a great balance of protein, carbohydrates, and fat.

Grab 'n' Go

Mojito Smoothie

This refreshing smoothie has the bright taste of lime and mint and is just creamy and sweet enough to be dessert-worthy.

Makes 1 serving

Serving size: 1 shake
Calories per serving: 165
Protein per serving: 21 grams
Carbohydrates per serving: 14 grams
Fat per serving: 4 grams

1 scoop Zen Fuze vanilla protein powder (or your favorite vanilla protein powder)

½ cup almond milk

½ cup water

Juice from ½ lime

Dash of lime zest

5–8 mint leaves

Stevia (optional)

Ice

1. Combine all ingredients in a blender until smooth.

What Is the Balance?

This recipe is a good balance of protein, carbohydrates, and fat, although the carb and fat totals are slightly low. If hungry, feel free to add a little extra fruit and nuts on the side for additional fat and carbohydrates.

Plant Based

Due to the high amount of carbohydrates found in most plant-based options, these plant-based recipes will be less balanced than the other recipes provided in this book. To boost your protein in these recipes, add a plant-based protein shot on the side. Some options for your protein shot are Vega One, Warrior Blend, or a low-fat hemp powder. Simply take a scoop of the protein powder, mix it in water, and drink it before or along with your meal. This will help balance out your meal.

Gourmet Style

Springtime Roll of Love

This is a fun vegan twist on the classic sushi roll. Fruit and nuts on the side help round out the meal. Nori seaweed is used to make sushi rolls and can be found in the Asian section of larger grocery stores. A trip to the local Asian market may be necessary if your grocery store does not carry it.

Makes 4 servings*

Serving size: 1 roll, approximately 1 cup fruit salad, approximately
   ⅓ cup nuts or seeds
Calories per serving: 401
Protein per serving: 15 grams
Carbohydrates per serving: 34 grams
Fat per serving: 28 grams

---

*Females have only half serving per meal.

4 sheets sushi nori roasted seaweed

1 cup sliced carrots

1 cup sliced snow pea pods

1 avocado, thinly sliced

2 cups broccoli sprouts

1 cup raspberries

4 clementine oranges, peeled and separated into wedges

4 small kiwis, sliced

½ cup chopped raw walnuts

¼ cup raw cashews

¼ cup raw almonds

¼ cup raw shelled pistachios

¼ cup raw pumpkin seeds

¼ cup raw sunflower seeds

1. Place a nori sheet on a moistened bamboo rolling mat.

2. Lay in sliced carrots, pea pods, avocado, and broccoli sprouts and roll according to directions.

3. Slice the roll and set it on a plate.

4. Mix fruit in a bowl and serve on the side.

5. Mix all nuts and seeds in a bowl and serve on the side.

What Is the Balance?

Add a plant-based protein shot from Vega One or Warrior Blend (or any brand that passes your protein powder litmus test explained in the Clean step of the Detox chapter and in the supplement reference section at the back of this book) or a low-fat hemp powder. Simply take a scoop of the plant-based protein powder, mix it in water, and drink before or along with your meal. This will provide a solid balance of protein, carbohydrates, and fat.

Eggplant Wonderland

This magical-looking eggplant will surprise you with its rich flavor.

Makes 4 servings

Serving size: 3 slices eggplant, 2 cups salad
Calories per serving: 279
Protein per serving: 15 grams
Carbohydrates per serving: 26 grams
Fat per serving: 14 grams

1 large eggplant

Splash of marsala cooking wine

Dried basil

Dried thyme

4 cups baby spinach

2 cups baby arugula

2 cups cherry tomatoes

2 cups chopped baby peppers

2 cups baby snow pea pods

¾ cup raw, shelled hemp seed

2 limes

1. Cut eggplant into 12 slices (¼"–½" each).

2. Lay slices in a large saucepan and sprinkle with marsala cooking wine.

3. Sauté on medium-low heat until soft, approximately 10 minutes.

4. Season with basil and thyme to taste.

5. In a large bowl, toss spinach, arugula, tomatoes, peppers, pea pods, and hemp seed.

6. Place the eggplant and salad on plates. Just before serving, cut each lime in half and squeeze over salads.

What Is the Balance?

Add a plant-based protein shot from Vega One or Warrior Blend (or any brand that passes your protein powder litmus test explained in the Clean step of the Detox chapter and in the supplement reference section at the back of this book) or a low-fat hemp powder. Simply take a scoop of the plant-based protein powder, mix it in water, and drink before or along with your meal. This will provide a solid balance of protein, carbohydrates, and fat.

———————

Your engine is ready to burn some fat! Dive into your plug-and-play Ignite plan, and as you rock these next three weeks, remember these three things:

- **Love your food.** If you don't like your food, you'll eventually quit. Use your recipes and spice up your food with approved herbs and condiments.

- **Have fun with your exercise.** Make it fun so you feel like you're not even working out. That's the type of exercise you want to be doing. The exercise suggestions in your Thrive phase and chapter 7 will help you with that too!

- **Remember, we all fall off plan.** If you fall off plan, get right back on with the next meal. That will ensure steady progress. Worst case, if something happens that derails you for more than three days, no worries; just reboot your plan by repeating your Detox phase.

Make your 8 Week Run strong and powerful—it's your time to take back control of your health. Next up is your Thrive phase, when you truly learn how to evolve your plan into a way of life. Get ready to Reprogram, Diversify, and Energize!

Quick Support Reminder

Remember to make your 8 Week Run with people just like you. Having support and living your plan with others provides you a three times greater chance to stay the course and permanently achieve your goals. To be part of the community, simply visit *www.WhyKidsMakeYouFat .com/Community.*

After Picture Note Reminder

Once you complete your 8 Week Run, remember to take your after pictures (front, back, and side). You definitely want to have the visual proof of what you accomplished, and seeing your transformation will be all the inspiration you need to continue living a healthier life, despite the demands of your busy day.

5

THRIVE:
Live Your Life

**Weeks 5–8 and Beyond:
Reprogram, Diversify, Energize**

You're making your 8 Week Run and are now in that magic space—that cool moment in time when everything just works, where results come, you're making a stand for yourself, and you know what's possible with your health. Before becoming parents, we experienced this magic space much more. We had our victorious moments, and of course they would pass, but we knew they would be back. In essence, our time was ours. As parents, our time and focus have shifted, and those moments we used to have seem to quickly vanish into thin air. As our kids grow and their interests expand, our magic space shifts to their special moments and victories. It's what being a parent is all about: giving yourself to your kids, creating opportunities, and empowering them to be their best.

I've coached thousands of parents at this exact space where you now sit—the halfway point of your 8 Week Run when you either thrive and continue making yourself a priority or the moment when you begin to lose ground and your hold on your magic space. Life begins to push back, focus is lost, priorities shift, and within a few months, your results have disappeared and you're left scratching your head wondering how it turned so fast.

I'm sharing this with you because this is reality, and right now it can go either way for you. The past 4 weeks were a push and a challenge for yourself as you lived in an all-in mode, and it was necessary to take your body to the next level. Now as you enter your Thrive phase, it's all about shifting into a progression mode. The definition of *thrive* is to make steady progress, to prosper and flourish. That's what this chapter and the rest of the book are about. From this point on, every ounce of information is designed to provide you with the tools to continue living in your magic space. To keep results coming, to include your family and friends, and to truly evolve your plan into a way of life.

This is exactly what Leyla Nava faced. For a chronic dieter with high blood pressure, losing weight wasn't her difficulty—keeping the weight off and her blood pressure in check was. Leyla passionately made her 8 Week Run and lost twenty-eight pounds, twenty-two inches, and three pants sizes. The big question for her now was, would she fall back to her old ways or stay in her magic space? Leyla remembered it was her eighteen-year-old son who originally inspired her to make her run. He wanted her to live longer and have a higher-quality life.

Leyla Nava

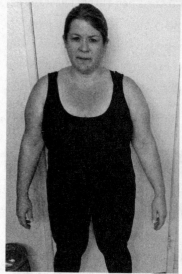

before

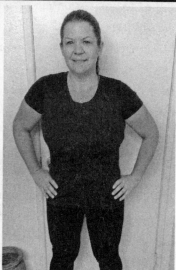

after 8 weeks

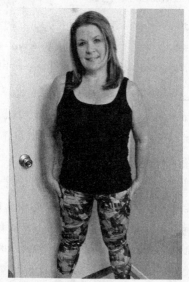

beyond 8 weeks

With that in mind, Leyla knew there was no going back. She shifted to progression mode and owned her Thrive phase. Seven months later (her 8 Week Run plus 5 months of Thriving), Leyla had dropped a total of fifty-three pounds, forty-four inches, and five pants sizes. What's even more exciting is she was able to stop taking her blood pressure medication! Now that's what I call a transformation inside and out.

► Your Three Thrive Result Options

Leyla's story is a great example of what's possible based on your goals and how progress can rapidly continue as you Thrive. This, of course, is unique to you and your goals, which is why there are three options to maximize your results during your Thrive phase. Please choose the one that relates best to you:

- You achieved your goals with your Detox and Ignite phases and are now shifting into a way of life. If this is you, you're ready for the full Thrive phase.

- You've had solid results and still have more to achieve. If this is you, keep living the Ignite phase for another 4 weeks, or do a hybrid version of the Ignite and Thrive phases. Just realize the more processed foods you work into your plan, the slower your results will come.

- You've made great progress in your Detox and Ignite phases but fell off plan multiple times. If this is you, repeat the Detox phase (seven days), and then shift into your Thrive phase. Depending on your goals, you may want to follow the Ignite phase guidelines or do a hybrid version of the Ignite and Thrive phases.

And once you've gone through the Detox and Ignite phases one time, you can then always do a hybrid version of all three phases. It's about evolving your plan so it works best for you, based on your goals and level of consistency.

---

3 Steps to Thrive: Reprogram, Diversify, Energize

Just as you saw in the Detox and Ignite phases, your Thrive phase is as easy as 1, 2, 3:

Step 1: Reprogram

Step 2: Diversify

Step 3: Energize

You reprogram your metabolism by staying consistent; you diversify your plan by adding in a weekly off-plan meal, new foods, and different exercises to prevent boredom; and you energize your new way of life by fully engaging your family and friends in the process.

▶ **Important Note**

In your Thrive phase, you will be following the same principles presented in your Detox and Ignite phases. Your plug-and-play Thrive meal plan will be presented at the end of this chapter along with your Thrive approved recipes.

Step 1: Reprogram

Think of a temperature-controlled room. It has a thermostat that maintains the temperature of the room. Let's say the temperature is set at seventy degrees. If the room goes above seventy degrees, the thermostat triggers the air conditioner to switch on and cool the room, and if the room goes below seventy degrees, the thermostat triggers the heater to turn on and heat the room. Just like the room has a temperature control system, your body has a weight control system, and they work almost identically. In your Detox phase, you lost your inflated weight, which got you back to the weight your body normally holds (or close to it). That weight was your true weight, meaning it's the weight your body typically gets stuck at. Your body's true weight is called your set point, and you have a weight-regulating mechanism (WRM) that works just like the room's thermostat. Basically, your WRM tells your body to burn or store calories in order to maintain your set point (true weight).

As you rocked your Ignite phase, you burst through your set point, lowered it, and now sit at a new weight. Your next step is to keep your momentum flowing long enough to actually reprogram your set point and metabolism to your new weight. Here are two steps to make sure your results and new weight are here to stay:

- **Stay consistent:** It sounds so simple, but after we push through the Detox and Ignite phases, it's easy to take a breath and begin to backslide. This is why your Thrive phase is so important, because it actually reprograms your metabolism. In this phase, you need to hold your new weight for at least two months. It takes about that amount of time for your body to recalibrate. You can of course keep dropping weight, inches, and body fat if you have more to lose—just remember, every step of progress forward needs to be followed by consistency for your results to stick.

- **Live in a five-pound range:** Yo-yo dieting is what kills your metabolism. Any big swing in weight loss followed by weight gain causes havoc in your body. As you thrive and evolve your plan, make sure you keep your weight within a five-pound range. For example, I have a client, Veronica, who lost thirty pounds during her 8 Week Run and her new weight was 140 pounds. She stayed consistent and reprogrammed her set point to that weight. At times she would have a tough week, go on a vacation, kids would get sick, and so on—basically things would cause her plan to be less than ideal—but she paid attention to her five-pound range. If she got to 145 pounds, she would immediately snap right back and tighten up her plan. It's unrealistic to think you can hold an exact weight for the rest of your life, but what you can do is hold a five-pound range. This provides you with the flexibility you need while also ensuring you have solid boundaries. If your goal is to continue losing weight, simply adjust your five-pound range for each new weight milestone you hit.

Step 2: Diversify

As you started your 8 Week Run, I promised you this time would come—the time when you get to add some of your favorite foods back in, including a little alcohol and coffee and of course a weekly off-plan (aka cheat) meal. Thriving is about shifting into progression mode, which means still moving forward, just at a more realistic pace.

Now, the more you diversify and expand your plan, always remember the lesson learned in chapter 1: your actions must match your expectations. Meaning, as you diversify and add additional foods to your plan, if your results are no longer coming as quickly as you want, then you may need to diversify a little less and do a hybrid of your Ignite and Thrive phases, or simply shift your goals. Either way, the key is to find the right balance where you feel you can truly live your plan for the rest of your life. To keep your plan exciting, you'll be adding more food choices to your daily meals, an optional weekly off-plan meal, and moderate alcohol and coffee (if you want), and you'll be expanding your workout boundaries to continue keeping your exercise fun and challenging. Let's start with your new tasty food choices.

New Thrive Phase Foods

Lean and Non-Lean Proteins

You already have a large variety of protein (there are just not a ton of different types of proteins), but I know these dairy additions are what many of you have been waiting for.

Warning! Dairy is still a bloating food, so be very cautious about how much you add back in, especially cheese. At best, add these moderately back into your plan and make sure that if you eat yogurt, it's Greek yogurt. Greek yogurt is processed differently than other yogurt, so it has more protein and much less refined sugar and lactose (the sugar found in milk that I shared earlier can cause bloating). Here's a snapshot of your new protein additions:

- Cheese (natural, minimally processed and low sodium)

- Cottage cheese

- Greek yogurt

> ## Quick Note

Feel free to experiment with all foods in your Thrive phase. Just follow the guidelines you've learned and do your best to choose foods with fewer than five ingredients on the label. This ensures the food is pretty clean. Obviously, the cleanest foods have one ingredient, like fresh meats, fruits, vegetables, raw nuts, and so on.

> ## Milk Note

For optimal results, natural and unsweetened almond is your best milk choice. If you choose to add cow's milk (dairy) back into your plan, do it moderately and make sure to adjust the carbs and fat in the rest of your meal to keep it balanced.

Grains / Calorie-Dense Carbs

In order to stop a revolt, it's time to bring back some of the most requested foods, bread and pasta. Just like with dairy, proceed with caution when adding additional grains back into your plan. Ideally, choose gluten-free and the most natural and unprocessed options. I love gluten-free brown rice pasta. It tastes great, doesn't bloat me, and keeps me on plan—a triple win! Here's a snapshot of your new grain options:

- Bread

- Couscous

- Hot cereal (Cream of Wheat, grits, and oatmeal; Ignite phase approved oatmeal is always your best choice)

- Pasta

Fats

The party just keeps rockin', especially with your new fat options. I know I might sound like a broken record, but remember, the more processed foods you add to your plan, the slower your results will come, so just keep that in mind. You're always much better off sticking to the list of fats in your Ignite phase and only sparingly adding these additional fat options. If you add them in, choose the least processed and most natural brands of each. Here's a snapshot of your new fat options:

- Butter

- Guacamole

- Mayonnaise

- Salad dressing

- Sour cream

Condiments

One of the great things about this plan is, after eight weeks your taste buds change and the salt and sweetness you used to crave with every meal just aren't so appealing anymore. With that being said, it's still important to have some additional condiment options in case you do want to add a sauce or to occasionally salt your food.

Here's a snapshot of your new condiment options, and you'll see salt is back. I'm a man of my word—I promised there would be a time when salt could be moderately worked back in your plan, and that time is now!

- BBQ sauce (low sugar)

- Ketchup (low sugar)

- Mustard (low sodium)

- Sea salt and/or pink Himalayan salt (if you want salt, only use these two options, both natural and unprocessed, but remember it's still salt, so keep it moderate)

Weekly Off-Plan Meal (Optional)

Let's face it—food tastes great. I love pizza, ice cream, doughnuts, fried chicken, hamburgers, french fries, etc. For me, this list could just keep going on and on. If I thought I would have to give up my favorite heavy-carb and high-fat foods forever, I would check out. Who wants to feel like they can't have something for the rest of their life? Not me! The reality is, almost everything added in moderation is fine, and by simply knowing that you can have your favorite foods, you actually want them less. Go figure.

In your Thrive phase, you can work in a weekly off-plan meal (aka cheat meal). Basically, you can eat anything you want for one meal a week. You read that right—one *meal*, not one day. I like calling it an off-plan meal because that's what you're doing, just going off plan for a moment. I'm not a fan of the term *cheat meal* because it sounds like you are doing something wrong.

When you go for it, here are some strategies to help minimize the damage (fat storage) of your off-plan meal and get you right back on plan:

- Eat in threes up until your off-plan meal so your metabolism stays active.

- Make your off-plan meal an experience, forget about all portion sizes, eat anything you want, and have fun—you earned it!

- Get right back on plan after your off-plan meal.

➤ **Quick Off-Plan Meal Note**

Your off-plan meal is optional. Depending on your goals, you may want to do one weekly, every two weeks, or monthly. Listen to your body, and if you really want an off-plan meal, go for it. Just keep making sure your actions (effort) match your expectations (goals).

Alcohol and Coffee

When you started your Detox phase, you might have been counting down the days to get alcohol and coffee back in your plan. Funny how things can change in eight weeks. Now that you've detoxed and your metabolism is on fire, you just don't crave the same foods and drinks anymore. With that being said, I know most people do enjoy an occasional glass of wine, cold beer, steamy cup of coffee, or shot of espresso. So if you're in the mood for some alcohol or coffee and want to stay on plan, here are your recommended guidelines:

ALCOHOL

- Limit yourself to one drink, a maximum of two times per week. Choose either a glass of wine (six ounces), a shot of hard liquor (vodka is your best choice because it's clear, which means it has fewer impurities and grit than other types of hard liquor), or a beer (twelve ounces, preferably light).

- Remove your grains and calorie-dense vegetables from your meal when you add alcohol with it. This helps minimize the damage (unwanted fat storage from the meal). Simply choose a protein, fat, and low-calorie veggie, and use your alcohol as your carb. For example, chicken (protein), salad (low-calorie veggies), avocado on the side (fat), and your alcohol choice.

COFFEE

- Limit to one to two cups per day.

- Avoid high-calorie coffee and tea drinks.

- If caffeinated, avoid drinking in the late afternoon/evening, as this can interfere with your quality of sleep.

> ### Quick Tea Note

You've been able to use caffeine-free herbal teas since you started your Detox phase, and you added green tea extract in your Ignite phase to assist with boosting your metabolism. Feel free to now add any caffeinated teas you enjoy. Simply follow the same guidelines listed for coffee.

Expand Your Exercise Horizon

You learned the three types of exercise in your Ignite phase, you've developed a weekly routine, and you have some solid fat-burning, high-intensity, and strength-training workouts. That's excellent progress! Maintaining your magic space is all about expanding your exercise horizon and testing your boundaries. The moment your workouts become boring or same old, same old, you're in trouble. Here are three strategies to keep your exercise fun, effective, and fresh:

- Each month, experiment with a new type of fat-burning cardio, high-intensity cardio, and strength training. For example, for fat-burning cardio, if you're currently only jogging or walking, experiment with cycling, swimming, or rowing. For high-intensity cardio, if you're only sprinting or spinning, take a kickboxing class or start cardio tennis. For strength training, if you're only doing Pilates or weight training, dive into yoga or a new class at your gym.

- Each month, as you diversify your exercise and test new types of workouts, some you'll like, some you won't. For the ones you like, rotate them into your workout routine.

- Each month, try a sport that provides you with the cardio you need but doesn't feel like you're working out. We all have different interests, so the variety of sports can vary greatly. Here are a few to give a shot—they work for all ages, and there might even be adult leagues in your area: tennis, paddle tennis, racquetball, squash, running (5K, half marathons, and marathons), basketball, soccer, swimming, cycling, triathlons, rowing, trampoline, and so on. Find the ones that pique your interest, and let the games begin!

Step 3: Energize

Growing up, I watched my mom and sister Laurie eat their low-calorie, cardboard-looking "diet" foods at dinner while my dad, my other sister Chris, and I were eating "normal" food. In the 1980s, this is what dieters thought they had to do. Eat less food, fewer carbohydrates, and no fat—basically starve themselves. My mom, who worked a full-time job as a nurse and had three children and a husband, came home exhausted each night and then needed to make two dinners, all because she thought that was the only way to not gain weight. I remember those nights like they were yesterday, wondering why it had to be like that. I hated seeing how hard it was for my mom.

In essence, those dinner nights back in the eighties are a huge reason I'm writing this book. Families shouldn't need to eat separately, parents shouldn't need to make two separate dinners, and families should be able to rock their health together. Your Energize step is all about making your plan a permanent part of your world and truly including your family and friends. There are three specific themes I'll introduce to get you started and make sure you continue to evolve this list. All families are different and have different interests, so make sure you evolve your plan to match your family's vibe.

- **Eat meals together.** What's so cool about your food plan and all the recipes in this book is that they're all about real food that is great for toddlers to grandparents and everyone in between. It's just clean, healthy, and balanced food. No cardboard-tasting meals here! Whether it's Abbi or me making the meal, it works for the entire family. I know we all live busy lives, so eating meals together does not necessarily mean sitting down together at the table to eat dinner (if you

can do that with your family, though, all the better—great
bonding time!). Eating meals together means making one
type of meal so the entire family can eat it, whether it's fresh
or as leftovers. This makes cooking, grocery shopping, and
the overall eating experience so much simpler. We all learn
by doing and we lead by example, so eating as one family
creates the healthiest food patterns for you and your kids. It
also develops excellent traditions for your kids to teach their
kids as they become parents.

- **Exercise together.** Growing up, I loved how my dad would
  always be up for a new game, whether it was football in
  the street, whiffle ball at the park, soccer at the field, or a
  quick game of tennis at the high school courts. My dad and
  I were always looking for ways to make exercise fun and,
  most importantly, to do it together. That's what exercising
  together is all about. Because my dad instilled these exercise
  traditions in me, it was already in my blood to do the same
  with Hunter. What's even cooler is that Abbi's dad also
  instilled exercising-together principles in her, so Hunter
  truly has the best of both worlds. Whether we go for a family
  hike, or we hit Sky Zone to play some indoor trampoline
  dodgeball (seriously one of Hunter's and my top sports in
  the world), or Abbi and Hunter take on an obstacle course in
  our basement (or at the park), or we all have an intense ping-
  pong battle in our living room, we find ways to stay active
  and exercise together as a family. We all know life is busy,
  and those past moments of slipping out and getting sixty
  minutes of exercise in by yourself are a bit more challenging
  as a parent. Working out together creates awesome family

time while fitting in your much-needed exercise time, knocking down two cans with one stone!

- **Live healthy together.** This concept goes hand in hand with eating your meals and exercising together. It basically means living your health with your family and your friends. The dinner example I shared, with my mom eating her diet foods, was just one of the many moments of separation she went through as a dieter. It was never about living healthier and together—it was about losing weight and the feeling that she had to suffer and alienate herself as a dieter. My mom never wanted that—she just thought that's what she had to do, like millions of other dieters. But it doesn't have to be that way. It's really as simple as joining a walking group, or sharing a recipe with a friend, or having a monthly clean cooking night in your neighborhood. These are just a few examples of how to live healthy together with your family and your friends, and the cool thing is, the more you do it, the more ideas will evolve and your initial spark of health will inspire your family, your friends, and your community.

Sherry Huva took the Energize step to a new level. Sherry and her family have always been health conscious and active, but as life continued to get busier, Sherry started noticing that her clothes became tighter and the mirror not as friendly. She also saw her family starting to lose focus on their health by eating out more and exercising less. Sherry dove full throttle into her 8 Week Run and in the process has become an incredible amateur chef. Her clean and balanced meals were so tasty that her family couldn't wait for dinner. Her new excitement about exercise motivated the rest of the family to get more active. And by leading by example, Sherry

Sherry Huva

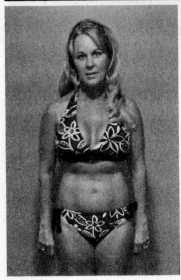

before

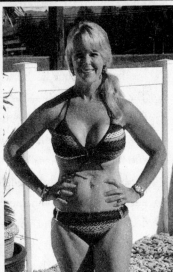

after 8 weeks

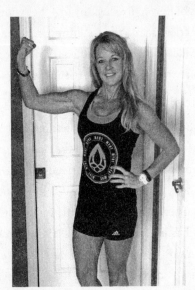

beyond 8 weeks

created an awesome environment for the Huva family to live their health together. Oh, and by the way, that mirror is back on great terms with Sherry. She dropped from a size 6 to a size 0/1. She made two 8 Week Runs and dropped a total of twenty-two pounds and ten inches.

You've got the concepts of Reprogramming, Diversifying, and Energizing, and now it's time to dive into your Thrive plug-and-play meal plan!

Your Plug-and-Play Thrive Plan

Your plug-and-play plan for the Thrive phase is on the following five pages.

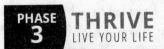

PHASE 3 THRIVE
LIVE YOUR LIFE

GUIDELINES FOR YOUR THRIVE PHASE

Important Note

In your Thrive phase you will be following the same overall principles as in your other phases, only you'll be adding some great variety and diversity to your food and exercise to permanently make your plan a part of your world.

> Repeat your Ignite phase weeks 5–8 and fat burning supplements if your goal is to still lose weight and maximize fat burning and start your Thrive phase beginning Week 9.

Guidelines to Optimize Your Portion Sizes (same as Detox and Ignite phases)

- ✓ Let go of the calorie mind-set. Simply follow the portion sizes and meal plan designed for your gender.
- ✓ You can measure your portion sizes by weight or with your hands (palm, fist, and thumb). Do whatever is easiest and most convenient.
- ✓ Make sure you're hungry (ready to eat but never starving) before each meal and satisfied (never full) after. If you're hungry before 3 hours, simply eat a balanced meal before the 3-hour mark.
- ✓ If you measure food with a scale, always measure it precooked since weight will be lost during cooking. If you measure portion sizes with your hands, always measure after it's cooked (only applies to cooked food).

Guidelines to Optimize Your Results:

- ✓ New meal guidelines for Thrive phase:
  - ⇒ Add new food options for protein, fat, and carbs to provide greater meal diversity for you and your family.
  - ⇒ You can shift to 1 shake a day if you prefer or keep it at 2 shakes (can use protein bar/RTD shake for convenience).
  - ⇒ Add a weekly off-plan meal (whatever you want and make it an experience), then just get right back on plan.
  - ⇒ If you add alcohol back in, limit it to 1 of these, max 2 times per week: glass of wine, 1 shot of hard liquor, or 1 beer. Make sure to cut all complex carbs from any meal where you drink alcohol.
  - ⇒ If you add in caffeinated coffee or tea, limit to 2 cups max a day.
- ✓ Keep eating in threes and follow the mealtime and water guidelines presented in this phase (Thrive).
- ✓ If you fall off plan for more than 3 days, you can reboot your plan by simply repeating your 7-day Detox phase.
- ✓ **Supplements are optional. They are designed to turbocharge your results.** ◆
  - ⇒ If your goal is to still burn fat, cycle Fat Burning Supplements ◆ 8 weeks on / 2 weeks off.

◆ Specific recommended brands of shakes, bars, & supplements can be found in the reference section.

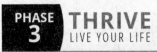

PHASE 3

THRIVE
LIVE YOUR LIFE

WEEKS 5-8 AND BEYOND

1 REPROGRAM

REPROGRAM your metabolism by keeping your momentum flowing.

It's easy to lose focus after taking your body to a new level, but to truly make your results and new weight permanent, you must keep your body moving forward, maintain a five-pound range and continue shifting your plan into a way of life.

SAMPLE MEAL PLAN
see next page for suggested meal portions + foods

Breakfast	Protein + Carb + Fat (Ex.: Egg Whites + Gluten-Free Bread + Peanut Butter) (with Essential Fats and Fiber Supplements) ◆
Midmorning	Protein Shake (with Digestive Supplements) ◆ OR Complete Meal (Ex.: Greek Yogurt + Blueberries + Cashews)
Lunch	Protein + Carb + Fat (Ex: Turkey Avocado Wrap)
Midafternoon	Protein Shake (with Digestive Supplements from list) ◆
Dinner	Protein + Carb + Fat (Ex.: Chicken + Gluten-Free Pasta + Salad w/ Tomatoes + Avocado) (with Fiber Supplements) ◆
Late night	Protein Shake ◆ OR Complete Meal (Ex.: Egg White Banana Pancakes) (this meal is optional, eat if hungry)

2 DIVERSIFY

DIVERSIFY your plan by adding an off-plan meal and new foods and exercises.

Boredom is the #1 culprit for falling off plan and starting to backslide.

To keep your plan exciting, you will:

- Add a weekly off-plan meal (aka cheat meal) *(this is optional)*

- Add more of your favorite foods (examples being Greek yogurt, gluten-free bread, and pasta) and moderate alcohol (if you drink)

- Add additional workouts to keep your cardio and strength training fun

- Add Zen Fit, an amino acid product designed to protect your muscle, assist with protein digestion, and help with reprogramming the overall speed of your metabolism.

3 ENERGIZE

ENERGIZE your new way of life by engaging your family and friends.

Ideally you included others in your 8 Week Run. If so, great job! If not, no worries. It's now time to truly make your plan a part of your world, and that's only possible by living it with others.

To energize your plan, you will:

- Eat meals together
- Exercise together
- Live healthily together

◆ Specific recommended brands of shakes, bars, & supplements can be found in the reference section.

PHASE 3 — THRIVE
LIVE YOUR LIFE

SPECIAL NOTE:
The same portion sizes and food exchange system guidelines in the Ignite phase apply to the Thrive phase.

PORTION EXCHANGE SYSTEM & RECOMMENDED FOODS

★ New to Thrive phase

PROTEINS	CARBOHYDRATES	FATS	FREE FOODS
PORTION SIZES	**PORTION SIZES**	**PORTION SIZES**	**PORTION SIZES**
FEMALES / MALES	FEMALES / MALES	FEMALES / MALES	NO LIMITS
1 Palm (3 ounces) / **1½–2 Palms** (5 ounces)	**1 Fist** (3 ounces) / **2 Fists** (5 ounces)	**1 Thumb** / **1 Big Thumb**	

CHOOSE 1 PER MEAL	CHOOSE 1 PER MEAL	CHOOSE 1 PER MEAL	UNLIMITED
✓Lean Proteins • Bison *(extra lean)* • Chicken • Egg Whites ★ Greek Yogurt *(fat-free)* • Hemp *(low in fat, ex. hemp powder)* • Lean Fish *(shellfish is now okay)* *(ex. tuna, halibut, tilapia, etc.)* • Turkey • Venison ✓Non-Lean Proteins *(do not choose additional fat w/ these proteins)* • Beef *(filet mignon)* • Beef *(ground 99% lean)* ★ Cheese *(natural)* *(use sparingly)* • Cottage Cheese *(low fat)* • Eggs, Whole • Fish *(non-lean)* *(ex., salmon)* ★ Greek Yogurt *(low fat)* • Hemp *(regular fat content)* • Lamb • Pork Tenderloin ✓Protein Powder *(shakes)* ◆ • Whey & Micellar Casein: Zen Fuze Shake *(made by Jeunesse)* • Hydrolyzed Whey: Proto Whey • Plant Based: Vega One or Warrior Blend • Egg White: Many Quality Brands	✓Fruits • Apples • Bananas • Berries • Grapefruit • Mangos • Oranges • etc. ✓Vegetables • Bell Peppers • Broccoli • Carrots • Cucumber • Squash • Tomato • etc. ✓Grains/Calorie-Dense Veggies [1] *(choose gluten-free when relevant)* • Beans *(choose fresh/dried)* *(ex, black, kidney, garbanzo, etc.)* • Bread • Brown Rice ★ Couscous • Millet ★ Oatmeal / Hot Cereals ★ Pasta ★ Potatoes *(sweet potatoes are best)* • Quinoa • Yams 1 For grains/calorie-dense veggies, use hand sizes rather than weight.	✓Avocado ★ Butter *(moderate)* ✓Chia Seeds ✓Flax Seeds ★ Guacamole *(moderate)* ★ Mayo *(moderate)* ✓Natural Nut Butters *(1 tbsp. for females)* *(1½ tbsp. for males)* ✓Oils *(½ tbsp. for females)* *(1 tbsp. for males)* • Olive • Coconut • Macadamia ✓Olives [2] ✓Raw Nuts *(½ oz. ~ small handful - for females)* *(1 oz. ~ medium handful - for males)* ★ Salad Dressing *(moderate)* ★ Sour Cream *(moderate)* 2 For olives, use hand sizes rather than weight.	✓Herbs • Basil • Bay Leaves • Cilantro • Dill • Parsley • Rosemary • Sage • Thyme • etc. ✓Spices • Cinnamon • Garlic • Ginger • Nutmeg • Peppercorns • Saffron • etc. ✓Leafy Greens *(fresh only)* • Collard Greens • Kale • Lettuce *(all types)* • Spinach ✓Natural Sweetener • Stevia ✓Condiments ★ BBQ Sauce *(low sugar)* • Extracts *(almond, vanilla, etc.)* ★ Ketchup *(low sodium)* ★ Mustard *(low sodium)* • Vinegars *(balsamic, red wine, etc.)*

◆ Specific recommended brands of shakes, bars, & supplements can be found in the reference section.

PHASE 3 — THRIVE: LIVE YOUR LIFE

SPECIAL NOTE:
Use this meal structure for the rest of your life and keep expanding your food options.

SUGGESTED MEAL PLAN

Thrive Meal Plan for Females

	1 PROTEIN	1 CARB	1 FAT	SUPPLEMENTS
	SERVING SIZE 1 PALM (3 OUNCES)	SERVING SIZE 1 FIST (3 OUNCES)	SERVING SIZE 1 THUMB	SEE BELOW FOR SUPPLEMENT SERVING SIZE
Breakfast	3 Egg Whites (or 3 oz. protein from list)	1 slice Gluten-Free Bread (or 3 oz. carbs from list)	1 tbsp. Peanut Butter (or choose 1 serving fat from list)	**Essential Fats ◆** • Omega-3 Fatty Acids: 3000 mg **Fiber** • Psyllium Husk: 5 g (~ 1 heaping tsp.) ‡
Midmorning	Shake ◆ or Meal Consisting of Protein, Fat, + Carbs (ex. Greek Yogurt, Blueberries, and Cashews)			**Digestive ◆** • Pro-Biotic: 1 capsule **OR** 1 Zen Fuze Shake **Muscle Protector ◆ ◇** • Zen Fit **Fat Burning ◆ ◇** (keep taking if goal is to still maximize fat burning)
Lunch	3 oz. protein	3 oz. carbs	1 serving fat	
Midafternoon	1 Shake Serving ◆ (serving size is based on nutrient label; for best results, use water. If needed can add up to ½ cup of unsweetened almond milk or coconut water)			**Digestive ◆** • Pro-Biotic: 1 capsule **OR** 1 Zen Fuze Shake **Muscle Protector ◆ ◇** • Zen Fit **Fat Burning ◆ ◇** (keep taking if goal is to still maximize fat burning)
Dinner	3 oz. protein	3 oz. carbs	1 serving fat	**Fiber** • Psyllium Husk: 5 g (~ 1 heaping tsp.) ‡
Late night	Shake or Meal Consisting of Protein, Fat, & Carbs *meal optional - eat if hungry* (ex. Banana Pancakes made with extra Egg Whites for protein)			

‡ Fiber Supplements are optional if having daily bowel movements. ◇ Take indicated supplements 30 min. before a meal.

Water Recommendations

2–4 Liters / Day

8–16 Glasses (8 oz.)

Drink water with each meal and between each meal.

◆ Specific recommended brands of shakes, bars, & supplements can be found in the reference section.

PHASE 3 **THRIVE** LIVE YOUR LIFE

SPECIAL NOTE:
Use this meal structure for the rest of your life and keep expanding your food options.

SUGGESTED MEAL PLAN

Thrive Meal Plan for Males

	1 PROTEIN	1 CARB	1 FAT	SUPPLEMENTS
	SERVING SIZE	SERVING SIZE	SERVING SIZE	SEE BELOW FOR SUPPLEMENT SERVING SIZE
	1½–2 Palms (5 ounces)	**2 Fists** (5 ounces)	**1 Big Thumb**	
Breakfast	5 Egg Whites (or 5 oz. protein from list)	2 slices Gluten-Free Bread (or 5 oz. carbs from list)	1½ tbsp. Peanut Butter (or choose 1 serving fat from list)	**Essential Fats ◆** • Omega-3 Fatty Acids: 3000 mg **Fiber** • Psyllium Husk: 5 g (~ 1 heaping tsp.) ‡
Midmorning	Shake ◆ or Meal Consisting of Protein, Fat + Carbs (ex. Greek Yogurt, Blueberries, and Cashews)			**Digestive ◆** • Pro-Biotic: 1 capsule **OR** 1 Zen Fuze Shake **Muscle Protector ◆ ◇** • Zen Fit **Fat Burning ◆ ◇** (keep taking if goal is to still maximize fat burning)
Lunch	5 oz. protein	5 oz. carbs	1 serving fat	
Midafternoon	1–2 Shake Servings (based on your level of hunger) ◆ (serving size is based on nutrient label; for best results, use water, if needed can add up to ½ cup of unsweetened almond milk or coconut water)			**Digestive ◆** • Pro-Biotic: 1 capsule **OR** 1 Zen Fuze Shake **Muscle Protector ◆ ◇** • Zen Fit **Fat Burning ◆ ◇** (keep taking if goal is to still maximize fat burning)
Dinner	5 oz. protein	5 oz. carbs	1 serving fat	**Fiber** • Psyllium Husk: 5 g (~ 1 heaping tsp.) ‡
Late night	Shake or Meal Consisting of Protein, Fat, & Carbs *meal optional - eat if hungry* (ex. Banana Pancakes made with extra Egg Whites for protein)			

‡ Fiber Supplements are optional if having daily bowel movements.   ◇ Take indicated supplements 30 min. before a meal.

Water Recommendations
3–5 Liters / Day
12–20 Glasses (8 oz.)

Drink water with each meal and between each meal.

◆ Specific recommended brands of shakes, bars, & supplements can be found in the reference section.

THRIVE
Approved Recipes

Here are your Thrive approved recipes with a bonus side dish and dessert section to keep your food exciting and bursting with flavor! Just like with your Detox and Ignite recipes, you can eat any Thrive recipe at any meal. Make sure to use recipes from all three phases to give yourself variety, and as with your other phases, your Thrive recipes will be labeled:

- **Grab 'n' Go:** 10 minutes or less, for when you're in a time crunch

- **Gourmet Style:** 30 minutes or less and perfect for a nice dinner with your family and/or friends

> ## Some Quick Recipe Reminders

Venice Nutrition Head Chef Valerie Cogswell and I oversaw the recipes. This collection is a mixture of recipes developed by Chef Valerie, Venice Health Professionals, and other 8 Week Runners just like you. Chef Valerie has also provided her top recipes for each phase—these recipes have two asterisks (**) by the recipe title.

The recipes are presented in the order of breakfast, lunch, dinner, shakes, and plant based. In this phase there is a bonus dessert and side dish section. The calories and macronutrient breakdowns (protein, carbohydrates, and fat) are listed based on serving size, and each recipe can be eaten anytime throughout the day. Follow the portion sizes presented in your plug-and-play meal plans, and remember to stay focused on eating in threes.

Each recipe features a balance section that either tells you the recipe itself provides the correct balance of macronutrients (protein, carbohydrates, and fat) or gives you the specific sides to eat along with the recipe to provide that balance. Easy to follow so there is no guessing!

Breakfast

Grab 'n' Go

Greek Yogurt Parfait**

Creamy, vanilla-sweetened, protein-packed Greek yogurt is layered between fresh berries and nuts in this mouth-watering parfait. You can easily make this recipe in bulk for quick meals all week long; just add the fruit and nuts right before serving. Greek Yogurt Parfait is a kid-friendly favorite and makes a sweet and simple breakfast, snack, or dessert. If you're in a hurry, you do not need to layer ingredients; just mix them all together.

Makes 1 serving

Serving size: 1 yogurt parfait and ¼ cup fruit
Calories per serving: 263
Protein per serving: 25 grams
Carbohydrates per serving: 21 grams
Fat per serving: 8 grams

10 ounces fat-free, plain Greek yogurt

½ teaspoon vanilla extract

Stevia

¼ heaping cup berries (raspberries, strawberries, etc.)

½ ounce nuts (pecans, almonds, walnuts, etc.)

1. Stir together Greek yogurt, vanilla extract, and desired amount of stevia.

2. Layer the yogurt mixture in a dish with berries and nuts. If you're in a hurry, simply mix all the ingredients together until combined.

What Is the Balance?

This recipe has a great balance of protein, carbohydrates, and fat.

Three-Minute Omelet with Mozzarella, Sweet Tomato, and Fresh Basil**

In a rush most mornings? This easy breakfast has a balance of complete protein, carbohydrates, and fat to help you burn fat and feel your best all day long. Best of all, this recipe takes only minutes to make in the microwave and has simple yet delicious ingredients like sweet grape tomatoes, fresh basil, and mozzarella cheese.

Makes 1 serving

Serving size: 1 omelet
Calories per serving: 177
Protein per serving: 22 grams
Carbohydrates per serving: 3 grams
Fat per serving: 7 grams

Fat-free cooking spray

3 egg whites

¼ cup shredded mozzarella cheese

Handful sweet grape tomatoes, sliced in half

Sea salt or pink Himalayan salt

Freshly ground black pepper

Fresh basil

1. Spray a microwave-safe bowl with fat-free cooking spray.

2. Add egg whites to bowl and cook in microwave for 1½–2 minutes, or until eggs are almost set.

3. Top with cheese and microwave another 30 seconds. Top with tomatoes.

4. Season with a pinch of salt and freshly ground black pepper. Garnish with fresh torn basil leaves.

5. Serve with a little fresh fruit on the side to make sure you're getting enough carbs.

What Is the Balance?

This recipe has a great balance of protein and fat. Please add a small amount of carbohydrates like fresh fruit on the side for a balanced meal.

Cottage Cheese, Apple, and Peanut Butter Bowl**

Low-fat cottage cheese, vanilla extract, natural peanut butter, and apple chunks are blended to sweet perfection.

Makes 1 serving

Serving size: 1 bowl
Calories per serving: 251
Protein per serving: 21 grams
Carbohydrates per serving: 20 grams
Fat per serving: 8 grams

6 ounces low-fat cottage cheese

3 ounces apples, chopped

½ tablespoon natural peanut butter (smooth or chunky)

¼ teaspoon cinnamon

¼ teaspoon vanilla extract

Stevia

1. Place first five ingredients in a blender and blend until smooth.

2. Sweeten to taste with stevia.

Note: For a chunkier version, mix it in a bowl instead of blending.

What Is the Balance?

This recipe has a great balance of protein, carbs, and fat.

Lunch

Gourmet Style

Chicken Salad with Dried Cherries and Honey Thyme Vinaigrette**

From the peppery arugula to the earthy, sweet dressing and tart cherries, this simple yet artfully prepared salad is sure to become a staple. For ideal preparation, make sure to use a nonstick pan when sautéing the chicken.

Makes 5 servings

Serving size: 3 ounces chicken with 2 cups salad
Calories per serving: 285
Protein per serving: 21 grams
Carbohydrates per serving: 20 grams
Fat per serving: 13 grams

FOR THE DRESSING

Juice from ½ lemon

½ teaspoon grainy Dijon mustard

4 tablespoons extra virgin olive oil

1 shallot, chopped

1 teaspoon chopped fresh thyme

1 tablespoon honey

½ teaspoon sea salt or pink Himalayan salt

Freshly ground black pepper

FOR THE CHICKEN

   1 pound chicken breast, cubed

   ½ teaspoon paprika

   ¼ teaspoon garlic powder

   2 tablespoons flour

   Sea salt or pink Himalayan salt

   Freshly ground black pepper

   Fat-free cooking spray

FOR THE SALAD

   7 cups arugula

   1 cup grape tomatoes, sliced in half

   ½ cucumber, diced

   ½ cup dried cherries

1. Pour lemon juice in a small bowl.

2. Whisk in mustard. Slowly whisk in extra virgin olive oil until combined. Whisk in remaining dressing ingredients.

3. Taste for seasoning and adjust as desired. Set aside to let flavors blend.

4. Toss chicken with paprika, garlic powder, flour, a pinch of salt, and a small pinch of pepper.

5. Heat a large, nonstick frying pan over medium heat. Once pan is hot, generously spray with fat-free cooking spray. Allow to heat for 2 minutes.

6. Add chicken and sauté about 6–8 minutes or until no longer pink inside, making sure not to overcook. Set aside.

7. Combine arugula, tomatoes, and cucumbers. Toss with vinaigrette.

8. Top dressed salad with chicken and dried cherries.

What Is the Balance?

This recipe has a great balance of protein, carbohydrates, and fat.

Gourmet Style

Spicy Turkey and Black Bean Chili**

This rich and spicy chili recipe is easy to make and great for family lunches or dinners and grab 'n' go meals all week long. Fresh toppings like sour cream, cilantro, and diced red onion add texture and flavor. Try doubling the ingredients for plenty of extra meals throughout the week. To increase the heat, add more cayenne pepper or jalapeño.

Makes 7 servings

Serving size: 1 heaping cup
Calories per serving: 258
Protein per serving: 20 grams
Carbohydrates per serving: 25 grams
Fat per serving: 7 grams

Fat-free cooking spray

1 (20-ounce) package 93% lean ground turkey

1 tablespoon plus 1 teaspoon cumin

1 teaspoon thyme

½ teaspoon sea salt or pink Himalayan salt, plus extra if necessary

½ teaspoon cayenne pepper

1½ teaspoons paprika

1 medium Spanish onion, chopped

2 stalks celery, finely chopped

1 small green bell pepper, chopped

½ jalapeño, finely chopped

4 large cloves garlic, finely minced

1 (28-ounce) can diced tomatoes (Cento brand petite diced is good)

1 (20-ounce) can black beans

½ cup light sour cream

1 small red onion or bunch of scallions, finely chopped

1 bunch fresh cilantro, chopped

1. Spray a pot with fat-free cooking spray and place over medium-high heat.

2. Once hot, add ground turkey and break up meat with spatula.

3. Add cumin, thyme, salt, cayenne, and paprika and cook until turkey is no longer pink, about 7 minutes. Once turkey is cooked, use a slotted spoon to remove it to a bowl (keeping as much fat as possible in the pot) and set aside.

4. Add onions, celery, and bell peppers to the pot and sauté for approximately 3 minutes.

5. Season gently with a pinch of salt.

6. Add jalapeño and garlic and continue to sauté for another minute.

7. Add turkey to the vegetables in the pot and stir well.

8. Add tomatoes and beans and simmer, covered, over low heat for about 15 minutes (or more if you have the time) until thickened.

9. Top with 1 tablespoon of sour cream per serving and some red onions and cilantro.

What Is the Balance?

This recipe has a great balance of protein, carbohydrates, and fat.

Barbecue Chicken Flatbread Pizza**

Sometimes nothing but pizza will do! This easy, flavorful pizza has a delicious balance of protein, carbohydrates, and fat to help you burn fat, build muscle, and feel your best. Cook chicken breast in bulk for the week for quick grab 'n' go meals like this one. Kids will love this recipe too.

Makes 1 serving

Serving size: 1 small pizza
Calories per serving: 280
Protein per serving: 23 grams
Carbohydrates per serving: 15.5 grams
Fat per serving: 11 grams

1 low-carbohydrate, 8″ whole-wheat or gluten-free wrap or tortilla

Fat-free cooking spray

2 tablespoons all-natural tomato sauce

⅓ cup reduced fat (not low-fat) sharp cheddar cheese, divided

2½ ounces cooked boneless, skinless chicken breast, cut into small chunks or shredded

1 tablespoon all-natural barbecue sauce

Onion, thinly sliced (optional)

Bell pepper, thinly sliced (optional)

1. Preheat oven to 450°F.

2. Place wrap/tortilla on a cookie sheet and spray the wrap/tortilla lightly with fat-free cooking spray.

3. Spread tomato sauce on top.

4. Sprinkle half of the cheese on top of sauce.

5. In a small bowl, combine the chicken and barbecue sauce, and then layer on top of cheese.

6. Sprinkle onions, peppers, and remaining cheese on top of pizza.

7. Cook for 8–10 minutes, or until crust is crisp and cheese is melted.

8. Allow to cool slightly, cut into quarters.

What Is the Balance?

This recipe has a great balance of protein, carbohydrates, and fat.

Dinner

Grab 'n' Go

Sautéed Shrimp and Quinoa**

Looking for a delicious and balanced dinner? Our Sautéed Shrimp and Quinoa is packed full of protein and fiber. Fresh herbs, olive oil, lemon juice, and tomatoes make a natural and flavorful sauce.

Makes 5 servings

Serving size: 4 ounces shrimp plus 1 cup quinoa/veggies
Calories per serving: 292
Protein per serving: 24 grams
Carbohydrates per serving: 30 grams
Fat per serving: 9 grams

- 1½ cups chopped raw green beans (tips removed)
- 2 tablespoons olive oil
- 1 shallot, finely chopped
- 1 heaping tablespoon chopped fresh thyme
- 1 pound raw shrimp, peeled, deveined, and tails removed
- 1–2 tablespoons plus ¼ cup low-sodium vegetable stock, divided
- Sea salt or pink Himalayan salt
- Freshly ground black pepper
- 1 pint grape tomatoes, washed and halved
- Juice from 1 small lemon
- 2½ cups cooked quinoa (follow instructions on the package)
- Chopped fresh parsley, for garnish

1. To cook green beans: Steam in the microwave for about 5 minutes or until al dente, or try blanching green beans to retain the color. To blanch green beans, fill a medium bowl with water and ice and set aside. Bring a small saucepan of water to a boil. Add green beans and boil for 3–4 minutes, or until al dente. Drain green beans and immediately plunge into ice water to stop the cooking process. This will help to retain the color of the green beans. Drain green beans and set aside.

2. Heat a large sauté pan over medium heat. Once hot, add olive oil.

3. Sauté shallots and thyme for 2 minutes, or until shallots are softened.

4. Add shrimp and sauté until pink, approximately 3 minutes. If pan dries out, add a couple tablespoons of vegetable stock.

5. Season gently with salt and pepper.

6. Remove shrimp and set aside. Return pan to medium heat.

7. Add tomatoes, fresh lemon juice, and ¼ cup of vegetable stock. Cook for 2–3 minutes.

8. Add green beans and cook for another 2 minutes.

9. Season gently with salt and pepper.

10. Add shrimp back to pan and sauté for about 1 minute to allow flavors to blend. Taste the mixture and add salt or pepper only if necessary.

11. Serve shrimp and vegetable mixture, including sauce, over quinoa.

12. Top with freshly chopped parsley.

What Is the Balance?

This recipe has a great balance of protein, carbohydrates, and fat.

Crust-Free Margherita Chicken Pizza

When you just want flavors of a fresh Margherita pizza, without the calorie- and carb-packed pizza crust, this version answers the call with minimal ingredients combined in the simplest of ways. Enjoy zesty pizza sauce, fresh mozzarella cheese, and fresh basil, tomato, and garlic, all served on top of a thin-cut crispy chicken breast (instead of regular pizza crust).

Makes 4 servings

Serving size: 1 chicken cutlet topped with ingredients (men get 1½ servings)
Calories per serving: 200
Protein per serving: 27 grams
Carbohydrates per serving: 5 grams
Fat per serving: 6 grams

- 2 large boneless, skinless chicken breasts
- Fat-free cooking spray
- ½ cup canned pizza sauce
- 4 ounces fresh mozzarella cheese, cubed
- 1 large tomato, diced
- Sea salt or pink Himalayan salt
- Pepper
- Garlic powder
- Red pepper flakes (optional)
- Parmesan cheese, freshly shredded
- Fresh basil

1. Preheat oven to 350°F.

2. Slice chicken breasts in half lengthwise to create a total of 4 thin chicken cutlets. Cover with plastic wrap and pound lightly with a food mallet into thin cutlets.

3. On the stovetop, brown chicken cutlets in a skillet sprayed with fat-free cooking spray for approximately 15 minutes or until crispy.

4. Spray a cooking sheet with cooking spray and place chicken on the sheet.

5. Top each chicken breast with approximately 1 tablespoon of pizza sauce.

6. Add 1 ounce of fresh mozzarella cheese to each breast and top with tomatoes.

7. Sprinkle lightly with salt, pepper, garlic powder, and red pepper flakes (if desired).

8. Bake for 15 minutes, or until the cheese melts.

9. Garnish with Parmesan cheese and fresh basil.

What Is the Balance?

This recipe is primarily protein and fat. Please add a veggie such as sautéed spinach or asparagus on the side for additional carbohydrates.

Gourmet Style

Zesty Thai Lettuce Wraps

Beat the boredom! Delicious and bursting with flavor, Zesty Thai Lettuce Wraps are a great idea for entertaining a group or serving a family-style meal! They can also be made ahead and reheated at any time.

Makes 8 servings

Serving size: 3 ounces cooked ground turkey/chicken
Calories per serving: 175
Protein per serving: 20 grams
Carbohydrates per serving: 6 grams
Fat per serving: 7 grams

Fat-free cooking spray

2 pounds 93% lean ground chicken or turkey

½ cup minced shallots or onions

4 ounces shredded carrots

½ cup thinly sliced red bell pepper

2½ tablespoons minced garlic

1 can chopped water chestnuts (optional)

2 tablespoons low-sodium soy sauce

2 tablespoons fish sauce (optional, omit for fish allergies)

4 teaspoons dark brown sugar

1 tablespoon Sriracha sauce (optional, can substitute red pepper

flakes for a no-sodium choice)

½ teaspoon freshly ground pepper

Iceberg lettuce leaves

Lime wedges

1. Heat nonstick, medium-size skillet over medium heat. Coat with fat-free cooking spray.

2. Add ground chicken/turkey and cook about 15 minutes or until browned.

3. Add shallots, carrots, bell peppers, garlic, and water chestnuts and cook about 15 minutes or until tender.

4. Add soy sauce, fish sauce, brown sugar, and Sriracha sauce or red pepper flakes, and pepper and cook for 5–10 minutes, or until tender and flavors are infused together.

5. Spoon the mixture into the iceberg lettuce leaves to make the wraps and garnish with lime wedges.

What Is the Balance?

This recipe is primarily protein and fat. Please add a veggie on the side for additional carbohydrates.

Faux-lognese over Spaghetti Squash

While everyone loves Bolognese sauce, it's laden with fat and calories. This version will satisfy your taste buds and keep your waistline in check. Prepare the spaghetti squash ahead of time by cutting it in half, removing the seeds, and roasting cut-side down at 350°F for 45 minutes, or until the flesh shreds with a fork.

Makes 5 servings

Serving size: 3¼ ounces beef plus 3 ounces squash and sauce
Calories per serving: 205
Protein per serving: 18 grams
Carbohydrates per serving: 12 grams
Fat per serving: 10 grams

15 ounces fresh tomatoes

4 ounces onion

3 cloves garlic, minced

1 tablespoon olive oil

1 ounce fresh parsley

1 pound 96% lean ground beef

Fat-free cooking spray

2½ tablespoons Mrs. Dash Extra Spicy Seasoning Blend

½ cup unsweetened plain almond milk

3 cups cooked spaghetti squash

Romano cheese (optional)

1. In a food processor, blend tomatoes, onion, garlic, oil, and parsley.

2. On the stovetop, brown the ground beef with fat-free cooking spray. Drain fat and add Mrs. Dash no-salt seasoning.

3. Add the tomato mixture to the ground beef; cook for 5 minutes on low heat.

4. Add the almond milk to the pan and cook for 2 more minutes.

5. Serve beef mixture over 3 ounces spaghetti squash per serving.

6. Garnish with a sprinkle of high-quality Romano cheese if desired.

What Is the Balance?

This recipe has a great balance of protein, carbohydrates, and fat.

Gourmet Style

Easy Chicken Vegetable Soup**

If you're a chicken soup fan, you will love this recipe. It's not only incredibly easy and quick to make, but it's really good for you too. This hearty soup is full of rotisserie chicken and traditional vegetables and is sure to warm the soul.

Makes 10 servings

Serving size: 1 bowl
Calories per serving: 176
Protein per serving: 17 grams
Carbohydrates per serving: 9 grams
Fat per serving: 7.5 grams

- 1 whole rotisserie chicken (find at any grocery store or local market in the bakery/deli section)
- ¼ cup olive oil
- 1 large white onion, finely chopped
- 6 large carrots, peeled and chopped on the bias
- 2 cups chopped celery
- Sea salt or pink Himalayan salt
- Pepper
- 8 cups low-sodium, all-natural chicken stock
- 4 cloves garlic, finely minced
- 4 cups spinach leaves or escarole, shredded or chopped in large chunks
- 1 tablespoon fresh thyme (or 1½ teaspoons dried thyme)
- 3 tablespoons fresh parsley (or 2 teaspoons dried parsley)
- Hot sauce

1. With a pair of disposable latex gloves, remove the skin from the rotisserie chicken and discard. Carefully remove the meat from the bones. Keep a close eye out for small bones. Chop the meat and set aside in a medium bowl. Throw away the bones.

2. In a large stockpot, heat olive oil over medium-high heat.

3. Add onions, carrots, and celery and sauté until soft and fragrant.

4. Season lightly with salt and pepper. If using dried herbs, stir in now.

5. Reduce heat to low and add chicken pieces, chicken stock, and garlic. Bring to a simmer.

6. Allow to simmer for approximately 20 minutes, or until vegetables are cooked and flavors are developed (taste it!).

7. Before serving, add the escarole or spinach leaves and allow to wilt. If using fresh herbs, add now.

8. Add a few dashes of hot sauce and season to taste with salt and pepper.

What Is the Balance?

This recipe has a great balance of protein, carbohydrates, and fat. You can also add a small amount of brown rice to the soup (keep brown rice separate and add right before serving) to increase the carbohydrate content and make a complete meal.

Shakes

Grab 'n' Go

Berrylicious Smoothie**

When you're craving something cold, creamy, and sweet, try our Berrylicious Smoothie. Loaded with lush berries, tangy yogurt, protein powder, and a touch of vanilla, this vibrant fruity smoothie will boost your metabolism while delivering a powerful antioxidant punch.

Makes 1 serving

Serving size: 1 shake
Calories per serving: 270
Protein per serving: 25 grams
Carbohydrates per serving: 25 grams
Fat per serving: 8 grams

- **½ cup unsweetened almond milk**
- **2 tablespoons low-fat plain Greek yogurt**
- **1–2 scoops Zen Fuze vanilla protein powder (or your favorite vanilla protein powder; serving size depends on label, focus on 25 grams of protein)**
- **¾ cup frozen mixed strawberries, blueberries, blackberries, and raspberries**
- **½ teaspoon vanilla extract**
- **Splash of water, as needed**

1. Place all ingredients except water in a blender and blend on high until smooth and creamy. If smoothie is too thick, add a splash of water and continue blending until you achieve your desired consistency.

What Is the Balance?

If you're using a protein powder that naturally contains fat, like we did, there is no need to add additional fat. If you are using a protein powder that is fat-free, please add a few nuts on the side to increase the fat content for a balanced meal.

Frozen Coffee Protein Smoothie**

If your daily routine includes at least one stop at your local coffee shop for a frozen Frappuccino, you'll love our Frozen Coffee Protein Smoothie. A blend of protein powder, French vanilla coffee, and a touch of yogurt give this shake its rich coffee flavor and creamy texture. With six times the protein and only a fraction of the sugar of a store-bought frozen coffee drink, our Frozen Coffee Protein Smoothie is a healthy pick-me-up that won't spike your blood sugar. Add a piece of fresh fruit on the side, and you've got a fast and nutritionally balanced breakfast to go.

Makes 1 serving

Serving size: 1 shake
Calories per serving: 220
Protein per serving: 27 grams
Carbohydrates per serving: 16 grams
Fat per serving: 6 grams

- 1–2 scoops Zen Fuze vanilla or chocolate protein powder (or your favorite vanilla or chocolate protein powder; serving size depends on label, focus on 25 grams of protein)
- ⅓ cup French vanilla coffee (very cold), regular or decaf
- 2 tablespoons unsweetened almond milk
- 3 tablespoons low-fat plain Greek yogurt
- ¼ teaspoon vanilla extract
- 5 ice cubes

1. Place all ingredients in a blender and blend until smooth and creamy.

What Is the Balance?

This smoothie has a good balance of protein and fat. It is recommended that you add a small amount of high-quality carbohydrates, like fruit, on the side according to your personal nutritional parameters for a complete meal.

Plant Based

Due to the high amount of carbohydrates found in most plant-based options, these plant-based recipes will be less balanced than the other recipes provided in this book. To boost your protein in these recipes, add a plant-based protein shot on the side. Some options for your protein shot are Vega One, Warrior Blend, or a low-fat hemp powder. Simply take a scoop of the protein powder, mix it in water, and drink it before or along with your meal. This will help balance out your meal.

Grab 'n' Go

Summer Rolls

This is a no-cook, snack-style recipe perfect for any season. Rice pancakes are thin sheets of rice flour used to make spring rolls and can be found in the Asian food section of most large grocery stores. If they are not available in your store, a trip to the Asian market may be necessary.

Makes 4 servings

Serving size: 4 rolls
Calories per serving: 275
Protein per serving: 9 grams
Carbohydrates per serving: 29 grams
Fat per serving: 8 grams

16 rice pancakes

2 cups sliced carrots

2 cups broccoli sprouts

2 cups sliced baby peppers

¼ cup raw sunflower seeds

¼ cup raw, shelled pistachios

1. Lay rice pancake flat after moistening per package instructions.

2. Lay a quarter of each of the remaining ingredients on one side and roll together.

3. Repeat for the other three rolls.

4. Serve immediately.

What Is the Balance?

Add a plant-based protein shot from Vega One or Warrior Blend (or any brand that passes your protein powder litmus test explained in the Clean step of the Detox chapter and in the supplement reference section at the back of this book) or a low-fat hemp powder. Simply take a scoop of the plant-based protein powder, mix it in water, and drink before or along with your meal. This will provide a solid balance of protein, carbohydrates, and fat.

Ultra Protein Muffins

Vanilla and pumpkin make this earthy treat the perfect snack! These muffins do not rise as much as traditional muffins. For this reason you may fill the muffin cups nearly to the top. You may also use a brownie pan. This recipe is vegan-friendly and gluten-, nut-, dairy-, and soy-free. The ancient grain flours in this recipe can be found in most grocery stores. Bob's Red Mill is a popular brand that most larger stores should have available.

Makes 12 large muffins

Serving size: 1 muffin
Calories per serving: 118
Protein per serving: 6 grams
Carbohydrates per serving: 17 grams
Fat per serving: 4 grams

    ½ cup amaranth flour

    ½ cup buckwheat flour*

    ½ cup teff flour

    ¼ cup chia seeds

    ¼ cup hemp seeds

    ¼ cup ground flaxseed

    ½ teaspoon sea salt or pink Himalayan salt

    1 ½ cups organic pumpkin (canned)

---

*Farinetta buckwheat flour from Minn-Dak Growers has almost twice the protein.

2 teaspoons baking soda

2 teaspoons vanilla

2 teaspoons cinnamon

¼ teaspoon ground cloves

½ cup organic applesauce

1. Preheat oven to 350°F and line a standard muffin tin with muffin cup liners.

2. In a large mixing bowl, combine all ingredients.

3. Scoop batter into muffin cups.

4. Bake for 20 minutes, or until the centers are firm and the tops start to crack.

5. Allow to cool for 5 minutes before serving.

What Is the Balance?

Add a plant-based protein shot from Vega One or Warrior Blend (or any brand that passes your protein powder litmus test explained in the Clean step of the Detox chapter and in the supplement reference section at the back of this book) or a low-fat hemp powder. Simply take a scoop of the plant-based protein powder, mix it in water, and drink before or along with your meal. This will provide a solid balance of protein, carbohydrates, and fat.

Six Bonus Recipes

A rich, homemade tomato sauce. An elegant yet easy green salad. A feisty and versatile salsa. Bring life to your everyday meals with these chef-made staple side dishes and sauces and a delicious strawberry piña colada dessert. Enjoy!

Grab 'n' Go

Easy and Elegant Green Salad**

If you're looking for a salad that takes only minutes to make but complements everything from seafood to beef and is elegant enough to impress, this recipe is for you. The key to achieving the best flavor with this salad is to use the highest-quality and freshest ingredients you can find. Crisp romaine lettuce (or your favorite kind of greens) is tossed in fruity extra virgin olive oil and a shot of tangy balsamic vinegar. Sea salt, freshly ground black pepper, and fresh slivers of pecorino Romano cheese are the perfect accompaniments to this simple and delicious salad.

Makes 4 servings

Serving size: 1 plate
Calories per serving: 167
Protein per serving: 2 grams
Carbohydrates per serving: 10 grams
Fat per serving: 12 grams

3 tablespoons high-quality extra virgin olive oil

6 tablespoons balsamic vinegar

8 cups cut romaine lettuce (or your favorite greens)

Sea salt or pink Himalayan salt

Freshly ground black pepper

Aged, high-quality pecorino Romano cheese

1. In a small bowl, whisk together olive oil and balsamic vinegar.

2. In a large bowl, toss dressing with greens.

3. Season to taste with salt and pepper. Toss again.

4. Divide salad onto 4 plates.

5. With a cheese cutter, slice approximately 1 tablespoon aged pecorino Romano cheese to place on top of each salad.

What Is the Balance?

This recipe has a great balance of carbohydrates and fat. Please add a lean protein such as shrimp, fish, or chicken on the side for a balanced meal.

Chickpea and Basil Salad**

Who knew a simple combination of chickpeas, chopped veggies, and fresh herbs could be so delectable? Try this easy yet flavorful side dish at your next meal or cookout.

Makes 7 servings

Serving size: ⅓ cup
Calories per serving: 164
Protein per serving: 0 grams
Carbohydrates per serving: 22 grams
Fat per serving: 6 grams

FOR THE DRESSING

1½ tablespoons extra virgin olive oil

3 tablespoons red wine vinegar

1 clove garlic, minced into a paste

Small pinch of cayenne pepper (optional)

Freshly ground black pepper

FOR THE SALAD

2 (28-ounce) cans chickpeas, rinsed and drained

1 medium red bell pepper, chopped small

1 very small red onion, finely chopped

Handful fresh basil, rough chopped

⅓ cup (about 10) fresh, high-quality kalamata olives, pitted,
   roughly chopped

1. In a small bowl, whisk together all ingredients for the dressing and set aside.

2. In a medium bowl, toss together chickpeas, bell peppers, onions, and basil.

3. Pour the dressing into the bean-and-vegetable mixture and toss well.

4. Gently fold in the olives (over-mixing will cause the olives to color the remaining ingredients, so make sure to add them last and to toss gently).

What Is the Balance?

This recipe has a great balance of carbohydrates and fat. Please add a lean protein such as shrimp, fish, or chicken on the side for a balanced meal.

Vegetable Salsa**

Vibrant chopped vegetables are tossed with loads of garlic, jalapeño, tangy lime, and fresh cilantro in this easy vegetable salsa. A spoonful or two adds color, texture, and flavor to grilled seafood, chicken, pork tenderloin, brown rice, your favorite veggies, and even salad.

Makes 17 servings

Serving size: ⅓ cup
Calories per serving: 39
Protein per serving: 0 grams
Carbohydrates per serving: 8 grams
Fat per serving: < 1 gram

1 cup frozen or grilled corn, room temperature

1 pint cherry or grape tomatoes, quartered

½ cucumber, peeled, seeded, and chopped

1 (12-ounce) can low-sodium black beans, rinsed and drained well

1 medium red onion, diced

3–4 large cloves garlic, finely minced

1 small jalapeño, seeded and finely minced (use more if you like your salsa extra hot)

2 teaspoons olive oil

Large handful fresh cilantro leaves, chopped

Juice from 1 lime (or 2 if you prefer)

Sea salt or pink Himalayan salt

Freshly ground black pepper

1. Combine corn, tomatoes, cucumbers, beans, onions, garlic, jalapeños, olive oil, and cilantro in a bowl. Toss well.

2. Squeeze desired amount of fresh lime juice over the top and taste. Add more if necessary.

3. Season to taste with salt and pepper.

4. Refrigerate at least 1 hour to allow flavors to blend.

What Is the Balance?

In the amount of the suggested serving size, this is a low-calorie recipe consisting of mostly carbohydrates. For a complete meal, please add a protein, fat, and a small amount of carbohydrates. An example of a balanced meal with this salsa would include grilled salmon (protein and fat) with vegetable salsa (small amount of carbohydrates) and a side of brown rice or vegetables (more carbohydrates).

Guacamole**

This traditional guacamole is packed full of fresh, bold ingredients like creamy, heart-healthy avocados, tomatoes, onion, garlic, jalapeño, and cilantro. Use guacamole to replace mayo in your favorite wrap or on top of chicken, fish, or salad. You can also customize your guacamole by adjusting the amount of garlic, onion, jalapeño, lime, and cilantro; have fun with it and make it your own!

Makes 12 servings

Serving size: 2 tablespoons
Calories per serving: 75
Protein per serving: 0 grams
Carbohydrates per serving: 4 grams
Fat per serving: 6.5 grams

4 ripe avocados, pitted and chopped

1 tomato, seeded and chopped

½ small red onion, chopped

1 clove garlic, finely minced

½ small jalapeño, finely chopped (optional)

Small handful fresh cilantro (or as much as desired), chopped

Juice from 1 lime (or as much as desired)

Sea salt or pink Himalayan salt

1. Gently combine avocados with tomatoes, red onions, garlic, jalapeño, and cilantro.

2. Add desired amount of lime juice and season to taste with salt.

3. Mash to desired consistency.

4. Taste again for seasoning and adjust as necessary.

What Is the Balance?

Guacamole is a heart-healthy fat. Please add a carbohydrate and protein to make a complete meal.

Homemade Tomato Sauce**

Who has time to simmer sauce on the stovetop all day? This rich homemade tomato sauce is full of high-quality ingredients and takes about 30 minutes to make, from start to finish. Use homemade tomato sauce to top chicken, white fish, and even your favorite vegetables.

Makes 18 servings

Serving size: ⅓ cup
Calories per serving: 65
Protein per serving: 0 grams
Carbohydrates per serving: 10.5 grams
Fat per serving: 1.5 grams

  2 tablespoons extra virgin olive oil

  ¾ cup grated onion

  2 tablespoons celery, finely chopped

  1–2 large cloves garlic, finely minced into a paste

  2 (28-ounce) cans crushed tomatoes (not from concentrate, like
     Cento's crushed tomatoes)

  Water (optional)

  Sea salt or pink Himalayan salt

  Black pepper

  1½ teaspoons sugar

  ½ cup packed fresh basil leaves, roughly chopped

1. Heat olive oil over medium heat. Once hot, add onions and celery, and cook for about 5 minutes. Add garlic and cook 1 additional minute.

2. Add crushed tomatoes and simmer for approximately 20 minutes (or longer if you have time to—it will deepen the flavor) over low heat. Add a little water if sauce gets too thick.

3. Add salt (we used about ¾ teaspoon sea salt), pepper, and sugar.

4. Taste and adjust seasonings as necessary.

5. Stir in basil and simmer for 5 minutes. Remove from heat.

What Is the Balance?

This recipe is mostly carbohydrates and should be served with protein and fat (and some extra carbohydrates on the side) for a balanced meal.

Strawberries with Piña Colada Dip

In the mood for dessert? Try Piña Colada Dip, a creamy concoction of protein-rich Greek yogurt, coconut extract, and fresh pineapple that pairs perfectly with strawberries. This recipe is ideal for your next party, breakfast, dessert, or any time of day. For best results, make sure to use ripe, fresh pineapple. To check a pineapple's ripeness, smell the bottom of it; if it's ripe, it will smell sweet. Also, when the skin of a ripe pineapple is pressed, it will yield slightly. You can also purchase fresh, cut pineapple chunks in the fruit section of most supermarkets.

Makes 4 servings

Serving size: 1¼ cups dip with 5 strawberries
Calories per serving: 244
Protein per serving: 22.5 grams
Carbohydrates per serving: 26 grams
Fat per serving: 5.5 grams

FOR THE DIP

32 ounces plain, low-fat (2%) Greek yogurt

1 cup finely chopped fresh, ripe pineapple

1 teaspoon coconut extract

5 or more packets of stevia

STRAWBERRIES

20 strawberries, stemmed, halved or whole

1. Combine yogurt, pineapple, and coconut extract, adding enough stevia to reach desired sweetness.

2. Serve with fresh strawberries.

What is the Balance?

This recipe has a great balance of protein, carbohydrates, and fat and is a complete meal.

You now have the tools to live in your magic space and thrive! The remaining chapters will set you up to win regardless of what gets thrown in your path. They will truly empower you to make your plan a permanent part of your world. It's time to dive into chapter 6, where you'll take on the food frenzy of being a parent and learn the secrets of how to make your food work in any situation!

► **Quick Reboot Reminder**

We all know life shows up. If you find yourself in a place where you fell out of rhythm with your plan for a few weeks or possibly months, always know you can simply reboot your plan by repeating your Detox phase and then shifting into your Ignite or Thrive phases, or doing a hybrid of both. The Detox phase gets your body cleaned up and ready for action after a bit of a health sabbatical.

➤ Quick Recipe Note

The past three chapters have provided you with an excellent selection of tasty Detox, Ignite, and Thrive phase recipes. These recipes set you up to win and keep your food fresh and interesting. As you continue to live your plan, it's important to keep expanding your food boundaries and taste buds. A great way to do that is simply visit *www.WhyKidsMakeYouFat.com/Recipes* for additional recipes provided by our community and culinary team designed to work seamlessly into your plan.

6

Food Frenzy

Imagine if you had a remote control for your life, just like in the Adam Sandler movie *Click* (of course without any of the consequences). You could hit the pause button and shelve the time challenges that currently exist, creating the space to go full throttle and rock your 8 Week Run. Then as you live your Thrive phase and evolve your plan into a way of life, you continue moving at a steady pace, take the world off pause, and simply hit the slow-motion button. Then finally, once your plan becomes a part of your world, you hit the play button and everyone joins you at the real speed of life. How cool would that be?! The ability to adjust everything to your pace and give you the necessary time to take a breath, plan, and execute your new way of health. We can all dream . . . but until that remote control is created, the reality is, as parents we will live in a daily food frenzy time crunch.

The word *frenzy* means a state or period of uncontrolled excitement or wild behavior, and it's a perfect word to sum up what happens each day in most of our households. Whether it's hustling before school to get breakfast in for you and your kids, or scrambling to keep healthy and balanced food options as you become a midafternoon shuttle service for after-school extracurricular activities (sports, music, drama, etc.), or you attempt to do a quick run into your local grocery store with a hungry kid and a five-minute event turns into a thirty-minute battle to get out of the store (I've been there many times!), or finding the time as you wrap up a busy day to make a dinner that's quick, clean, and tasty for the entire family. Then after all that, you still need to feed yourself and find ways to make your food work. It's no wonder so many parents struggle with their health.

As you've seen, this book is all about making life easier for you and your family, which is exactly why you have your plug-and-play Detox, Ignite, and Thrive meal plans, along with delicious family-friendly recipes. Those tools already set you up to win. This chapter is all about providing additional cool ways to bring calmness to your food frenzy without the need for a remote control. It's time to create real solutions for the most challenging times to keep your food balanced and on schedule, which are grocery shopping ("Food Shopping Shakedown"), driving ("Taxi Service Syndrome"), and traveling ("On the Road Again").

Food Shopping Shakedown

For years every time Abbi and I went to the grocery store with Hunter (together or by ourselves), we felt like we were being hustled. Abbi and I called it a shakedown because from the moment we entered the grocery store, everything became a negotiation with Hunter and sometimes even a bribe! It's quite comical, especially because Abbi and I remember the pre-Hunter days, when we would watch families in a store and say, "Wow, when we have kids, there is no way we will give in to them like those parents." Ha! Exactly what every nonparent says. It was so naive of us, classic newbies, not having any clue about the shakedowns that occur every day by millions of kids or about the high-level negotiating skill set parents must possess to prevent the dreaded bribe.

I humbly admit that Abbi has always been so much better than I am at not caving in to Hunter's demands. It seemed Hunter had me under a spell and regardless of my stance or allotted time frame, by the time I would leave the store, he had everything he wanted. I would load the car with the groceries a bit shell-shocked wondering what had just happened. *How was I hustled again?* Eventually, with a little nudge from Abbi, I realized it was time to put a stop to this nonsense and create simple strategies that would set me up to win.

I watched how Abbi shopped with Hunter, used my knowledge of the body's physiology, and understood how grocery stores are designed. With all that information, I created three strategies to prevent the food shopping shakedown and help all parents, once again, be back in charge at the grocery store.

Now, we all know grocery stores have evolved into much more than just stores to buy food. There are endless adventures around every corner, including gadgets, toys, and distractions with each step. These three strategies will assist you not only in keeping the foods you buy clean and high quality but also in preventing your cart from filling up with lots of miscellaneous items kids love to buy!

Strategy 1: Never Shop Hungry— You or Your Kids

Think of when you're hungry. All foods look a little tastier, and your mouth begins to water even more for your favorite carbohydrates (cookies, candy, doughnuts, chocolate, bread, chips, etc.). This is straight physiology. When you're hungry, your blood sugar is getting low and your body is physically craving sugar for energy.

If you're grocery shopping by yourself and you're hungry, you possess the mental willpower to avoid the temptation of buying those carb-loaded foods (at least some of the time). But kids don't possess that same willpower. When kids are hungry, it's about a hundred times worse because their physical needs and wants overpower everything—they just want to eat, and all rationale is thrown out the window. Just remember a time when your kids were hungry and you went grocery shopping with them, and think of everything they wanted to eat and everything they asked for. Now think of a time when they weren't hungry and you took them grocery shopping—they most likely wanted and asked for less. Once you get the simplicity of how your body fuels itself, you'll immediately see that the number-one strategy in most situations is to never be very hungry (as I shared in earlier chapters, your goal is to be ready to eat when it's mealtime).

Your solution for this strategy is easy—just make sure you and your kids have a balanced meal before you go shopping. It can be a grab 'n' go meal, gourmet style, or a shake. Just follow the food guidelines based on the phase you're in, and your kids can use the food list from any of the phases. This strategy will set you up to win, and it will prevent all wandering food eyes at the grocery store.

➤ **Cool Tip**

This same concept applies when you're making meals with all the yummy food you bought at the store. We're classic food pickers, and most of the time the early nibbling is because we're hungry. So remember to start preparing your meal before you're so hungry that the picking and nibbling can't be stopped. And if you are having a hard time controlling yourself, simply have half a shake or protein bar to tide you over until the meal is ready.

Strategy 2: Have a Plan

The invention of the big-box grocery stores has changed the shopping experience from simply going into the store and buying some food to now feeling like the moment you walk through those electric sliding doors, you've entered an amusement wonderland. Colorful balloons lightly swinging in the air, the powerful aroma of fresh flowers, perfectly presented crisp and juicy seasonal fruits and veggies, cool and new gadgets labeled *Special of the Week,* and the intoxicating smell of just-out-of-the-oven baked breads, muffins, and pies. Seriously, how can we ever get upset with kids when they are drawn in with such fun and exciting options in the amusement wonderland of grocery stores?

What I realized is that since grocery stores have a plan, which is to create an experience for customers so they buy more stuff and keep coming back to shop, I needed to get on the offensive and create my own plan to counter the magical lure of the grocery shopping experience. Now you might be thinking, *Mark, I don't think of the grocery store as an amusement wonderland,* and I get that completely. Most adults don't, but kids do, and the best way to avoid the dreaded long, unwanted grocery store trips is to have a plan. Here are three simple tips to get your shopping plan started, and then you can continue evolving your plan to work for you and your family:

1. **Make a list of the proteins, carbohydrates, fats, spices, herbs, and condiments you want to buy that week.** You can write your list on a piece a paper or use the note section on your smartphone. Simply list what foods you want in each category, and focus on just buying enough fresh food items to last one week. Nothing is worse than wasting money because your food spoils.

2. **Shop the store's "battle map."** You've probably heard to shop on the outside aisles of the store, and overall that's a great concept. Ninety percent of everything Abbi and I buy is from the outside aisles, and that's where most of the unprocessed and natural foods are located. Whatever type of store you shop in, most of the foods you want to buy will be sectioned like this: first, fruits and veggies and many times healthy fats (avocado, raw nuts), followed by fresh meats and fishes, and then eggs and dairy (milk, Greek yogurt, cottage cheese, etc.). These items will be in the outer U shape of the store. The next section you'll visit is the natural section found in most stores. Go there to buy the rest of your dry goods like quinoa, brown rice, and gluten-free pasta. And finally, based on your list, you may need to enter the "war zone," which is the middle of the store. I call it the war zone because once you start aimlessly walking down aisles, you're in danger of a kid grenade going off and shopping time immediately shifting to negotiating time. To avoid a kid grenade, learn the aisles of the stores you shop in and know where the additional items you need like herbs, spices,

balsamic vinegar, and tea are located so you can go straight there and get right back out. This keeps you from entering the full war zone.

3. **Set a weekly grocery shopping schedule.** The fastest way to fall off plan and start scrambling for food is to let your refrigerator empty out. Being proactive is everything in keeping your food frenzy in check, and having a locked-in weekly grocery schedule goes a long way in maintaining calmness in your home. I also get that life as parents is unpredictable, so manage that by simply having a two-day window for weekly shopping. Abbi and I shop every Saturday or Sunday, depending on what we have going on that weekend. This way we have the flexibility between two days, but we always make sure we take on the week with a fully packed refrigerator, and in the rare times we don't, we know the week's food frenzy mode will be in overdrive.

Strategy 3: Choose Foods with Five or Fewer Ingredients

As you've learned in your Detox, Ignite, and Thrive phases, eating clean and unprocessed foods will deliver the most optimal results both internally and externally. So if possible, always buy organic, hormone-free, and gluten-free foods, as they will be your cleanest foods. As I briefly mentioned in your Thrive chapter, to make your food selection even easier, the simplest concept for you to follow and teach your kids is to look at ingredient lists. Basically, any food that has five or fewer ingredients is relatively clean. Your best choices are always foods with one ingredient, like fresh fruits, veggies, meats, and fish, as they are preservative-free. The more ingredients in a food, the more processed it is and the more junk it has to cause bloating and digestive challenges in your body. This makes five or fewer an excellent starting point and solid rule to follow when shopping. Then, based on your goals, you may even want to adjust to three or fewer ingredients or even only foods with one ingredient. That's completely up to you; base those decisions on your goals and the foods that help you realistically live your plan.

Taxi Service Syndrome

Back in 2003, two years before Hunter was born, a client walked into my office with a huge smile on her face.

I said, "Jane, you seem in great spirits today."

She replied, "Mark, I'm so happy. Finally, my last daughter just got her driver's license, and I'm no longer her taxi service!"

Fast-forward many years, and I'm now so clear on what Jane was talking about. In 2003 I understood what Jane was saying, but I wasn't living what she was saying—big difference. I had no idea that being a parent would add a new job to Abbi's and my résumés— owner and operator of a taxi service. As parents we live on the go and our kids need rides everywhere: school, sport practices, friends' houses, movies, and so on (the list never ends). And the crazy thing is, the older our kids become and their interests continue to expand, the more we have to drive.

Always being on the go makes it very difficult to keep healthy and balanced food options available, which leads to our cars becoming an extension of our kitchen tables, and many times fast food is the meal of choice. Well, unfortunately, I can't solve the taxi service addition to your résumé (that will naturally resolve itself when your kids become driving age), but I can definitely help with setting you up to win with a realistic mobile food system that keeps you on plan and out of the fast-food drive-through. I like to call the system your MRFK, which stands for mobile readiness food kit. Just like how your car has a roadside emergency kit (or it should, at least) for those unforeseen roadside challenges, your food plan needs an MRFK to help you navigate through those tough meal-times in the car.

Each family's MRFK varies a bit based on their individual goals and food choices, but there are some core essentials that everyone needs (just like how every roadside emergency kit has its core essentials like jumper cables, flares, tire patch kit, and so on). Here are the five core essentials to build your MRFK:

1. **Cooler:** Get a high-quality cooler that matches your style and is made to last. I suggest getting a couple, just in case there's a food explosion in one cooler (which happens more than you'd think). Then you always have a backup. A brand I love and use daily is Six Pack Bags. They have many styles for both men and women, and they're supercool because they have a built-in Tupperware carrying system.

2. **Reusable ice packs:** Get a few of these that match the size of your cooler. Too many times, after a long day, you forget to put the ice pack back in the freezer and then the following day, no ice pack (total bummer). The simple solution is to buy a few extras so you always have backup.

3. **Stainless steel containers, Tupperware, and airtight sandwich baggies:** Use high-quality Tupperware that fits well in your cooler and doesn't leak. Leaking Tupperware is

the main culprit of food explosions. Also, get some airtight sandwich baggies for all loose items such as protein powder, nuts, and supplements. And if you want to seriously take it to the next level, go the stainless steel route. Klean Kanteen makes portable stainless steel containers that keep food hot or cold for hours, and since they are stainless steel, you don't need to worry about any possible toxins that plastic can give off and possibly seep into your food.

4. **Water bottle and shaker:** Choose water bottles that are leak proof and easy to use. We all love the smell of some nice mildew from water spilling in our cars . . . not! Plus, kids love to throw water bottles on the floor, so a nice leak-proof one prevents all spillage. Ideally, have a couple extra water bottles for backup—it's easy to forget them in stores, so remember where you bring them (I've lost count of the number of bottles I've lost). My favorite water bottle brands are CamelBak (high-quality plastic) and Klean Kanteen (stainless steel). Both brands are extremely durable and high quality, and they have awesome locking systems that prevent spills. Also add a shaker bottle to your kit. Shakes are fantastic grab 'n' go meals. My favorite brand of shaker bottle is BlenderBottle— top-quality plastic and the best no-spillage shaker on the market (just make sure the lid is fully closed). And a big plus is they have multiple colors, so kids love them too!

5. **List of your favorite grab 'n' go food items:** Here are a few examples to help you get started:

   - **Proteins:** hard-boiled eggs, fresh turkey slices, tuna (extra-low sodium), Greek yogurt (only in Thrive phase), all natural and nitrate-free turkey jerky (only in Thrive phase)

- **Carbohydrates:** fresh fruits and vegetables

- **Fats:** nuts, hemp seeds, and avocado

- **Shakes, bars, and RTDs (ready to drinks):** Use the recommended brands in the reference section, or if you choose a different brand follow the litmus test shared in your Detox and Ignite chapters to ensure it's a quality product that matches your parameters.

To make your MRFK easiest to manage, keep a consistent stash of your favorite nonperishable foods—like nuts, protein powder, bars, and RTDs—in your cooler, and then each day before your taxi service begins, throw in fresh foods such as meats, fruits, and veggies.

Having your grab 'n' go list creates excellent clarity on the foods you can grab in a jam, but you can also prepare gourmet-style recipes and put them in your MRFK. Just always remember to eat in threes every meal. Keep evolving your list based on your goals and taste buds.

► **Quick Tip**

Your MRFK should also be used any time you're out of the house for more than a few hours, a few examples being shopping at the mall, running errands, or going to a kids' birthday party.

On the Road Again

Picture this: Abbi, Hunter, and I are running through the airport to catch our flight. Hunter's hungry (which was our first mistake!) and sees, but most importantly smells, Wetzel's Pretzel—pretzels that are so good, the word *pretzel* just doesn't do them justice. Hunter stops in his tracks and smoothly steps in line. Abbi and I are then forced to immediately put the skids on and backtrack to get Hunter. Abbi says, "Hunter, let's go. We don't have time." His reply of course is "I'm starving!"

Immediately, I knew we were in trouble and there was no point to argue. We had made the crucial mistake I shared in the "Food Shopping Shakedown" section—letting Hunter get too hungry. Fortunately the line moved quickly, but not as quickly as my heartbeat and the beads of sweat dripping down my forehead caused by the thought that we might miss our flight for a pretzel. Hunter got his pretzel (which was an unbalanced meal!), Abbi's and my stress levels normalized, and we luckily made our flight.

As you can see, stuff happens, meals can be missed, food mistakes made, and when you're on the road, everything is just harder. There's no "perfect" in any of our days. The more we move away from the semi-controlled comfort of our homes and kitchens, the easier it is for food mishaps to occur, and they will always happen. The key is learning from them when they happen, honing your skills, and being better prepared the next time you're in that same situation. This sets you up to win rather than scramble and stress. The airport example I just shared could have easily been avoided if we'd just made sure Hunter had a quick grab 'n' go balanced meal from our MRFK on the car ride to the airport.

Whether you're on a road trip, in an airplane, on a vacation, or taking a business trip, you can always win with your food by following these three easy strategies:

1. **Always have your MRFK.** Simply follow the same guidelines I shared in the "Taxi Service Syndrome" section. My motto: never leave home without it!

2. **Find a local grocery store and have a refrigerator in your hotel room.** When you're traveling you'll have food options at your hotel and local restaurants, but that only covers you for a few meals each day. I know that when Hunter comes with us on a trip, his appetite seems to double and he wants to keep snacking. The best way to keep those options healthy and balanced is by following the tips I shared in the "Food Shopping Shakedown" section. Those tips will let you walk into any grocery store, follow your list, shop efficiently, and check out quickly and easily. In addition, make sure to request a refrigerator in your hotel room. It's cool that most rooms now come with it, but just to be safe, when you make your room reservation, specifically ask for one. It's typically free of charge or at most a very minimal daily rate, which is worth every penny to stay on plan.

3. **Follow five guidelines to order in restaurants.** Whether you're out for healthy fast food, are going cafeteria style (like a buffet), or are enjoying a sit-down restaurant, the key to remember is you're in charge when ordering in restaurants. Here are your five restaurant strategies:

   • **Never arrive hungry.** You can see this theme just keeps recurring. As I've shared, we just don't think clearly or rationally when we're hungry. My buddy Mike was on vacation and caught a baseball game with his family. Unfortunately, he forgot to bring his MRFK, and after going six hours without food (he didn't want to eat the processed stadium food), he was starving. After the game, he and his family went to a restaurant, and the first thing he did was reach for the big loaf of bread and butter it up. That was a pure low–blood sugar moment, and his heavy-carb, high-fat, and calorie-loaded party just kept on rockin', all because he went to the restaurant starving. The first lesson Mike learned was to bring his MRFK in the future. But secondly, if he found himself in the same situation, he had learned he would be better off eating something, even if it's not balanced, than skipping a meal. He could have had some peanuts or a hamburger "animal style," which is just the meat patty in a lettuce wrap at the baseball game. Both of those options would have been much better than not eating.

- **Decide if you are on plan or off plan.** Now, sometimes you just want to go for it and let the food festivities rock on, which is exactly what your once-a-week off-plan meal is all about as you enter your Thrive phase. If you want to go for it and have an off-plan meal, take it on with your eyes wide open and make an experience out of it. Afterward, just get right back on plan. Nothing's worse than letting low blood sugar make the decision for you, which is exactly what happened to Mike in the example just shared. Mike felt guilty about his meal because it was a reaction to being very hungry, not because he officially wanted an off-plan meal. If you decide you're eating on plan, the next three strategies will help you keep the meal balanced and your progress flowing.

- **Choose your protein first and follow your recommended portion sizes.** Your protein choice will determine the rest of your meal. For example, if you choose salmon or steak, both have protein and fat in them, which means when you're on plan, you need to avoid all additional fat in your meal and move on to your carb choices. If you want some fat options in your meal, like balsamic vinaigrette or avocado on your salad or maybe some butter on your potato (if you're in the Thrive phase), then you need to choose a lean protein like chicken, turkey, or any white fish. Your protein choice sets up the rest of your meal, and then you choose your fat (if you're eating a lean protein) and then a carbohydrate (like rice, quinoa, or asparagus), and then simply follow your recommended portion sizes. Most restaurants provide extra-big serving sizes, so many times you can make two meals out of one. Simply get a box to go and eat the other half of your meal three to four hours later. Another excellent reason why you need a refrigerator in your room!

- **Order all sauces and dressings on the side and say no oil or added salt.** The worst reputation a restaurant can have is dry and flavorless food. For this reason most dishes will have extra sauce, oil, and salt. It's important to realize *you* are the boss! Restaurants want you to be happy and want your business, so when you order an on-plan meal, simply ask for all sauces and dressings on the side so you control how much goes on your dish. Also ask for your meal to be cooked without oil and added salt.

- **If you are going to have alcohol, cut the grains and calorie-dense veggies (complex carbs).** In your Thrive chapter, I shared how to moderately add alcohol back into your plan, and it's worth repeating the highlights. Basically, if you're in the mood for a cold beer or a glass of wine with dinner, simply cut the grains or calorie-dense veggies from your meal. Just have a protein (ex., halibut), a fat (ex., avocado), a light vegetable (ex., salad, broccoli), and a glass of wine or a beer or a shot of hard liquor, preferably vodka.

► **Quick Tip**

Through the years one of the biggest concerns my clients share is the feeling they are being too demanding when they order in restaurants and that they should just eat the food the way it's being made. My advice to that is simple: remember, *you are the boss* and you have goals that you want to achieve. Eating in restaurants is a part of life, especially with kids, and you need to take control of what you order to make sure it works for you and takes you closer to your goals. By implementing the strategies I just shared, your orders will be clean, simple, and easy for any cook to prepare. Plus, the more you order this way, the better you'll get at it. I can now order in any restaurant without even looking at the menu. I simply ask if they have chicken (my favorite protein), then if they have balsamic vinaigrette (my favorite dressing), a house salad (my leafy greens), and then quinoa or brown rice or sweet potatoes (my complex carb). Whichever one they have, I get it, and if for some reason, they don't have a clean complex carb, I double up on the veggies. Then when the food comes, I simply follow my portion sizes. You can do the exact same with your favorite foods. And one more quick reminder:

most restaurants now offer clean, gluten-free, and low-calorie dishes. Ask yourself why. It's because customers started ordering the way I just explained and restaurants knew they had to evolve to keep their business. Always remember, you're the boss!

There you have it, your plan to manage and minimize the food frenzy of life and especially as a parent. It's time to bring a little more calm into each day, which is exactly what Mark Timmerman needed to get his health back in order. Mark was a typical family man and businessman who worked hard and was always spending extra hours at the office when he should've been making more time for his health. His business dinners, travel schedules, and day-to-day chaos caused any focus on his food and exercise to be too overwhelming. This was when his wife, Kelly, stepped in.

Kelly was a cancer survivor and had always been health conscious. She knew if Mark was going to make his 8 Week Run and conquer his food frenzy, then she needed to lead the way. Kelly showed Mark that he didn't have to suffer and that he could still eat on the road, have a steak at a restaurant, and actually do realistic workouts that he would enjoy. Slowly and steadily, Kelly made Mark a believer, and what he once thought might be torture was becoming the highlight of his day. His new healthy habits were something he did with Kelly and their kids, and his mood, blood work, stress, and sleep all improved.

Mark and Kelly's results are incredible. Together they lost seventy-seven pounds and forty-one inches by making their 8 Week Runs and living the Thrive phase. And as Mark shared, one of the perks of his new look is he now actually gets checked out at the grocery

Kelly Timmerman

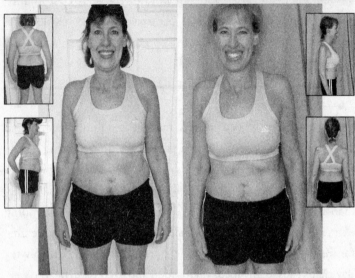

before

after 8 weeks

Mark Timmerman

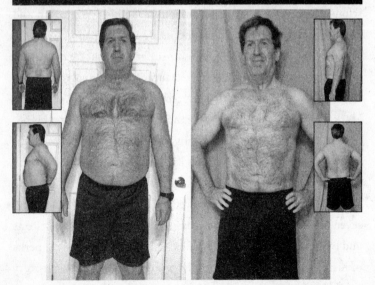

before

after 8 weeks

Kelly & Mark Timmerman

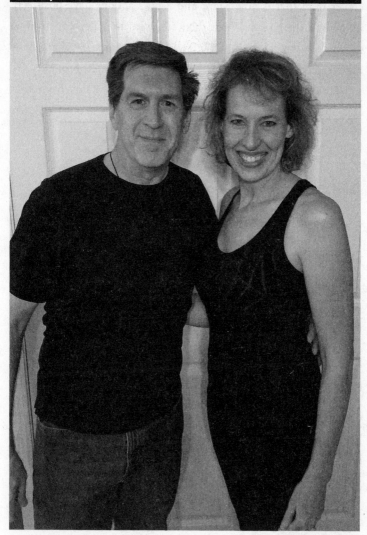

beyond 8 weeks

store by other women, always a confidence booster! But what's even cooler than that is how Mark and Kelly's actions have positively influenced their kids. When their son went to college, instead of gaining the typical freshman fifteen, he came home for Thanksgiving break fifteen pounds lighter simply by eating in threes.

Here's a super-quick recap and your action items from this chapter so you never need a remote control to pause or slow down life!

Take Control of the Food Shopping Shakedown

- Never shop hungry.

- Have a plan.

- Choose foods with five or fewer ingredients (one ingredient being best).

Keep Your Food Healthy and Balanced in Your Role as a Taxi Driver

Create an MRFK (mobile readiness food kit) in your own style. There are five main types of things you need for your MRFK (and keep expanding the list as you customize it):

- Cooler

- Reusable ice packs

- Tupperware and airtight sandwich baggies

- Water bottle and shaker

- List of your favorite grab 'n' go foods

Know You're the Boss of Your Food On the Road

- Always have your MRFK. Never leave home without it.

- Wherever you travel, if possible find a local grocery store and stock up on healthy and balanced foods. Also make sure you have a refrigerator in your room.

- Use these five guidelines when eating in any restaurant:

  1. Never arrive hungry (starving).

  2. Decide if you're on plan or off plan.

  3. Choose your protein first.

  4. Order all sauces and dressings on the side and say no oil or added salt.

  5. When adding alcohol, cut the grains and calorie-dense carbs (complex carbs) from your meal.

These strategies will greatly help you stay on track with eating in threes, which means your stored fat keeps steadily being released and burned up in your muscle for fuel.

In your Ignite chapter, you learned the three types of exercise, plus an exercise structure and parameters to optimize your workouts. Then in your Thrive chapter, you got some cool ideas on how to diversify your exercise and keep it fun. Now in chapter 7 it's time to address the time-crunch challenges with exercise we all experience as parents. Sometimes instead of going to the gym, you simply need to bring the gym to you. That's what chapter 7 is all about, bringing the gym to you and discovering the secrets of how to make your exercise happen anywhere and everywhere. Get ready to steal back your exercise time!

> ## Quick Info and Food Frenzy Support Tip

As your life evolves and stays busy your search will continue for additional strategies and ideas to master your food frenzy. For this reason, there's more food frenzy support through blogs, webinars, coaching videos and our online community. Simply visit *www.WhyKidsMakeYouFat.com/FoodFrenzy*

7

It Looks Like a Gym to Me

I t was a beautiful Sunday afternoon, and after three hard-fought soccer games, Hunter's U9 (under nine) team made it to the tournament final. As the boys warmed up for their final match, each parent could feel their own nervousness and intensity levels rise in anticipation for the game. The whistle blew, and sixty minutes of nonstop action and thrills began. With every pass, tackle, save, shot, and goal, each parent sitting—or, for those like me, standing—on the sidelines felt fully engaged and part of the competition. With only five minutes left, our team was winning 2–1, and we each looked at one another in agony, wondering how long five minutes could last . . . it felt like an eternity. Then, finally the referee blew his whistle, the match was over, and the boys ran to each other with their arms in the air, celebrating like champions.

As the boys celebrated on the field, all the parents were on the sidelines high-fiving each other and of course hugging it out (I love to hug)! After a few minutes of on-the-field and sideline celebration, we headed over to the award ceremony and watched each player receive a medal, followed by our awesome coach, JJ, sharing a few inspiring words about every boy. Then it was time to really get the celebration rolling, and the entire team went to our favorite restaurant to eat in style and cap off the championship weekend with a bang.

Experiences like these are what Abbi and I love about being parents—seeing kids flourish, excel, and build their confidence. In essence it's what being a parent is all about, providing every opportunity for our kids to succeed and become their very best.

But, as with everything great and meaningful, there can be a cost. The example I just shared shows how each parent was 100 percent connected to the moment and match—the only problem was that we didn't get the activity and exercise in like our kids did. We of course celebrated like we'd played, and many of us felt like we'd played (at least mentally), but in actuality, we didn't play. We basically *watched* all weekend and wrapped it up with a nice and hearty off-plan meal. This is the cost that every parent runs the risk of paying every day. The time we used to spend on our own exercise becomes hard to squeeze in, and the last thing we want to do is miss moments like Hunter's big win.

So, unfortunately, as parents we unknowingly become watchers. We watch our kids play and practice their sports. We watch our kids ride their bikes, play at the park, swim at the pool, and so on. The list of things we watch our kids do is endless. In the prekid days, we used to be the ones doing the activities, burning the calories, and having fun, but because of a true lack of time and a shift in priorities, we have morphed into calorie-storing watchers. Time becomes almost impossible to find, and if we can't get to the gym for sixty minutes, we think, *What's the point?* Well, it's time to abandon the watcher mind-set and realize that everywhere your kids are exercising, you can too. In essence, everywhere you go, with or without your kids, can become a gym.

In your Ignite and Thrive chapters, I shared ways to create a steady and consistent exercise plan and additional ideas on how to keep your workouts fun and fresh while involving your family and friends. Now it's time to take it to the next level and really address the main exercise challenge we have as parents: time. There just aren't enough hours in the day, so you end up stuck choosing between giving your kids the time they need and taking the time for yourself.

Well, picture being able to have both. Think of how cool that would be to have the quality and quantity of time with your kids while ditching your *watcher* label and getting back to being a doer. To steal back your workout time everywhere you are.

You see, there are three main places—these are actually better categorized as types of activities—where most of us spend our time: at work (office or home), involved in extracurricular/lifestyle activities (for your kids and yourself), and at home (typically after work and the extracurricular activities). If you calculate how many hours each day you're engaged in those three places, it's probably close to twenty-four hours (crazy to think we spend most of our time in three types of places!). Imagine stealing back your exercise time in each of those places; finding creative ways to burn extra calories, shed body fat, and tone your muscle without having to choose between being with your kids or taking that time for yourself.

Well, get ready because your time stealing starts now. Let's begin by turning your daily ho-hum work environment into some at-work adventures—in sixty seconds or less.

At-Work Adventures: Sixty Seconds or Less

Whether you physically go to an office, have a home office, are a stay-at-home parent, or a combination of all of the above, we all know that as parents we live in a constant state of time chasing—always trying to squeeze in as much as possible before our day shifts to the next responsibility and place we need to go. We feel this time pressure build throughout the day, so we hunker down, compartmentalize the best we can, and get our work completed. It becomes difficult to justify taking back any time for ourselves, especially knowing all the things we have on our to-do lists.

I totally get it, and I live it with you each day. What I had to realize is that once I get in my work zone, there's just no way I'm stepping away for thirty to sixty minutes to exercise because it would break the pattern and flow I'm in. It's just too big of a chunk of time, but I always go back to my motto of 1 percent.

I knew it was possible to steal moments of time throughout the day and turn stressful and inactive working hours into fun and physically effective working hours—without compromising my work but actually becoming more productive! Your at-work adventures are cool ideas and tips that take up sixty seconds or less and simply take things you're already doing each day and put a new spin on them to help strengthen your core (abdominals and lower back), increase your calorie burning, keep you hydrated, and create some peaceful and calm moments throughout your day.

Here are my five top adventures to get you started, and of course, as with every tip and strategy in this book, keep adding new ones to your list that are customized to you.

1. **Who needs a chair?** Think of all the times you sit throughout the day. If you add up that time, it would probably be equivalent to hours. By simply replacing your chair with an inflated burst-proof exercise ball, you will burn approximately three times as many calories per hour. Simply use the ball as your new chair, keep your back straight and shoulders back, activate your core muscles, and bend your knees for balance, and you have the most portable and effective chair on the market. And remember, it's all about 1 percent. No need to throw your chair out— sitting on an exercise ball may take some getting used to, so simply start with doing it for five to ten minutes per day and work your way up. Eventually it will become the only chair you need or want!

> ➤ **Quick Tip**

If you sit at a desk, make sure to check with a local fitness store to choose the size of exercise ball that is best for your body, which is primarily determined by your height.

2. **Climb away:** We all know we should use the stairs instead of an elevator or escalator—that's not a secret. But let's take that concept and multiply it by two. Basically, whenever you can take the stairs to your destination, double your trip, meaning go down and up twice in a row so you walk the

stairs two times. This will take less than sixty seconds and will add some extra cardio to your day. When you double your stair adventure, focus on keeping your core tight (back straight, abdominals contracted), pumping your arms (like you're marching), and contracting your thighs and glutes as you walk up and down the stairs (for some extra toning).

3. **Sixty-second bursts:** Set an alarm on your phone or watch for every hour. When the alarm goes off, immediately burst into sixty seconds of a strength-training movement. You can hold a squat, do desk push-ups, dive into a plank, pump some bicep curls, or sport some calf raises—basically whatever strength-training movements you are in the mood for, hit one for sixty seconds and then get back to work. You'll see that once you start doing this, your coworkers will want to join in on the fun and it will become an hourly event.

4. **Water cooler time:** Every hour go to the farthest water station in your office or house and fill up your bottle. If you only have to fill up a drop's worth of water, then you know you're not drinking enough, so drink up! By choosing the farthest station, you get some extra cardio in and your blood flowing. Then as you increase your water drinking, your bladder will start to fill up faster, and the outcome is more bathroom breaks, which equals more cardio—a double win! And if you have options, make sure to choose the farthest bathroom from your office for some extra cardio too. You may even get to climb away on some stairs too. Just keep remembering to keep your core tight and back straight as you march through each water cooler break.

5. **Zen moments:** You'll be amazed that simply spending sixty seconds stretching while listening to your favorite relaxing song can change your day. Every couple hours throughout your workday, simply put on your headphones, play one of your favorite songs, and stretch it out. Maybe you stretch your hamstrings, your lower back, or your neck. The combination of the music with some nice stretching will get you in full Zen mode and bring some much-needed peace and calmness to your busy day.

There you go, five simple and easy sixty-seconds-or-less at-work adventures. That's what's cool about stealing back your time—you just need to get creative and think outside the box. Your exercise moments are all around you at work, so just focus on the 1 percent moments. When you add those moments up, they make a huge difference.

After work and as the day moves on, most of us dive into some extracurricular and lifestyle activities like kids' practices, playground time, or possibly catching a movie. These activities have tons of exercise possibilities, so it's always game time. You just need to check your shyness at the door and realize this is your best time to steal back tons of workout time.

It's Always Game Time

Think of all the places you spend your time between working and hanging around your house—all those places are grouped as extracurricular and lifestyle activities. Now envision the endless possibilities of exercise in each of those places. You're as powerful as your imagination, and the more creative and spontaneous you can be, the sooner you'll see that it's always game time wherever you are. That's the magic of kids—they're always open and looking for an adventure, ready to turn anything into a spectacular extravaganza and start playing, regardless of the scenario. We were all kids and once had that same desire for fun, but with the pressures of life, the fear of looking silly, and the concern with what others might think (never even knowing who the others are), we've lost that spark we had as kids. So instead of playing, we continue to maintain our label as watchers. Well, no more.

It's time to once again activate your spark, start playing, and understand that it's always game time everywhere you go—you just need to be ready. I'm going to help get your imagination juices flowing with three real-world examples of how you can turn your normal daily activities that currently provide you with zero exercise into moments where you can steal back big chunks of bonus workout time. Let's dive in.

You Don't Need a Track to Walk

Typically Hunter's soccer practice is at a big grass complex with multiple fields. There may be six to eight teams training at once, and it's interesting to watch. Every boy and girl is out training hard and working up a sweat, and 99 percent of the parents are sitting in their chairs talking with each other and watching the activity. Then one day, our practice session was moved to a different complex, one that had a track. What happened during practice blew me away. About 40 percent of the parents who had been sitting in their chairs at the grass field bypassed their chairs and walked or jogged the track. It initially took me by surprise, and I then realized that most of us simply adapt to our surroundings. Because there was a track and an official place to exercise, it made sense for many of the parents to get active. But we all could've been walking or jogging even at the facility without the track.

In essence, that's what this chapter is all about: everything can be turned into a gym or exercise moment—you just have to visualize how to do it. Not needing a track to walk is a theme that transcends to all places, whether you're at a field, a park, a swim meet, basically anywhere you or your kids go. Instead of sitting and watching your kids be active, you get active too. You can do fat-burning cardio like walking or jogging, or maybe you dive into some high-intensity cardio like sprints or jumping rope. Bottom line, bring some sneakers, dress for a workout, and get to it. Soon you'll be keeping your chair in the car!

Hunter's elite soccer coach, JJ Gregoire, is a perfect example of this. JJ came to me and shared how he wanted to get back in shape. He used to be a big-time soccer player, and to the eye of the beholder, he still looked fit, but he knew that once the clothes came off or he did some sprints, he was far from it. I think we all know that feeling. JJ's son, Kiki, who also plays on the team, became his motivation. JJ wanted to do more activities with Kiki and start playing competitive soccer again, but it was tough. He was struggling to find the time and energy. He was on the field coaching teams or doing private lessons all day, six to seven days a week.

I coached JJ on exactly how to manage his food frenzy at the field and steal exercise time between team practices and private trainings. Now, you might be thinking, *Well, that's easy. He's already at the field,* but it's the exact opposite. Being at the field all day makes it harder to want to work out in that space, but when time is tight, you've got to do what you need to do. JJ took action, made his 8 Week Run, and got back into top shape, dropping twenty-one

JJ Gregoire

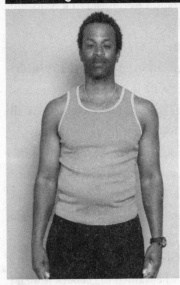

before

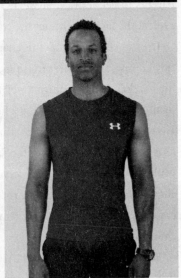

after 8 weeks

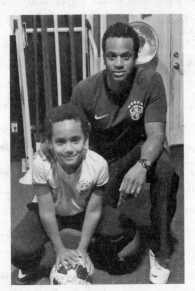

beyond 8 weeks

pounds and eighteen inches. And most importantly, he's got his energy back, is playing competitive soccer again, and has become a role model for Kiki and every player on Hunter's team and their parents on how to make your health happen!

Playground Social Hour

I remember when Hunter was a toddler, he would love going to the playground. Every time we drove in the car, he was on the lookout for a fresh new playground to hit up, his little eyes watching everything we passed, ready to yell, "Daddy, stop! I found a playground!" We would make our playground escapades fun and interactive, a cool game of tag, a swing competition, or even some pull-ups off the monkey bars. As we all know, playgrounds are also full of benches, designed for parents to sit, watch, and talk, and I must admit, if I was tired those benches were calling my name to just take a seat or possibly lie down and chill.

Your playground time all comes down to a choice, and you can simply shift the time you're spending on sitting and socializing to immediately switch it up into a fun-filled, intense workout. You can focus on tightening your core as you slide, or contracting your arms and legs while swinging, or getting some quick bursts of interval training in with a game of tag, or even squeezing some strength training in by lifting your kids a few times up and down. What's supercool is you get your workout in and you get to play with your kids. It just doesn't get better than that.

Looks Like a Sport to Me

My sister Laurie and her husband, Craig, have four kids, and their entire pack of six and our pack of three (Abbi, Hunter, and I), along with my mom and dad, all went to an amusement park together. This park had one of those fun houses where you can shoot foam balls at each other (so much fun!). When we walked into the building, we saw nonstop action and kids playing everywhere. And then of course all the benches, aka parent resting places, were full of parents sitting and watching.

It's like we become trained as parents—as our kids go and play, we're sectioned off to the bench area. Well, that's not how my family rolls. The moment Hunter and his cousins dove into the ball-shooting and throwing festivities, we grown-ups all rocked the house with them. We spent an hour running, sliding, throwing, and most important, laughing. Then after sixty minutes of fun-filled activity, all of us winded and sweaty, we were ready to hit some more roller coasters. We took a game of foam ball designed for kids and made it a sport for all of us to play—and that's what this example is all about, taking any activity and making it a sport.

Another great example is what Abbi, Hunter, and I do before we see a movie. We head to the movie theater a little early, and we bring our sneakers and a bouncy dodgeball, and we rock a twenty-minute game of wall ball (where you kick the ball off the wall to each other). This all started because we were waiting for a movie once and Hunter wanted to play. He saw a wall in the corner of the complex and started kicking his ball at it. Hunter looked like he was having fun, so Abbi and I joined in, and our sport of movie theater wall ball was born!

All these examples of game time are just a start for you to reactivate your spark, and they show you how easy it can be to shift from watcher status into doer status and steal back tons of exercise time. Wherever you go, all you need are some sneakers, workout clothes, a ball (any type), your imagination, and of course the willingness to let go of the attachment to what other people think. At the end of the day, choose to be different and do what's best for you and your family, and you'll soon realize it's a lot of fun knowing that it's always game time!

You have your at-work adventures set, new ideas to make your extracurricular and lifestyle activities game time, and now it's time to wrap it all up with turning your home into a fitness fun house!

Turn Your Home into a Fitness Fun House

It was a Friday night. I had just flown back home from a business trip, unlocked the side door, and as I came into the house, I was immediately hit in the chest with a Nerf bullet. I'd walked into the middle of a Nerf gun battle between Abbi and Hunter, and fortunately I survived it. Once I got hit, I immediately started laughing, and that moment instantly reminded me of how much I love that Abbi and Hunter always turn our home into a fitness fun house. Those two are always up for an adventure and looking for new ways to make our time at home fun, active, and interesting.

Typically after a long day of work and extracurricular activities, most of us feel like checking out and getting some much-needed downtime. Of course we all need our downtime, but many times you can simply replace some of your downtime, aka TV time, with unique exercise time. This chapter's theme is all about your creativity and ability to live outside the box and steal back your much-needed exercise time as a parent.

We all look at our home as our castles. Let's expand the title *castle* and add *fitness fun house* to it as well! Regardless of the size of your house, your home is an endless cardio and strength-training station for you and your kids. There are countless ways you can elevate your heart rate, tone your body, and keep your exercise fun. Here are some ideas and examples to get the exercise carnival rocking at your house.

- **Bounce city:** You can have a big trampoline in your backyard or a small one in your house—either way, bouncing on a trampoline is just fun. There's something so cool about jumping up and down that makes you smile. Besides the joy of jumping, trampolines are awesome exercise for your entire body and especially your core. Plus, jumping for three minutes straight helps clean out your lymphatic system (your body's drainage system).

- **Obstacle course Friday:** Just like how Abbi and Hunter played a Nerf gun battle, you can turn your home into an obstacle course or simply play a game of tag. Choose one night a week (or more) and replace a portion of your TV time with an obstacle course. You can make a few stations and time each member of the family to see who can master the course the fastest. Your course can be robust or simple (it depends on the size of your house and the sports equipment you have). It can be as easy as making four stations:

  Station 1: Weave in and out between four to six chairs two times forward and back.

  Station 2: Jump back and forth over a pillow ten times.

  Station 3: Hold a squat for sixty seconds.

  Station 4: Sprint around the room five times (or choose a different activity for this station if you don't like running in your house).

Then the family member with the best time wins, or you can do relays or multiple heats. Make it fun and keep thinking of new ways to make the course more challenging and exciting.

- **TV and movie experience:** You may not like movies or watching TV, but I love both! The challenge of course is time—where do I find it? In my home office, I have my road bike set up on an indoor bike trainer with my TV in front of my bike. This way, if my time is too tight to hit the tennis court or play some indoor dodgeball with Hunter or take our dogs for a walk, I can spin it out on my bike while watching one of my favorite movies or shows. The entertainment value prevents the boredom of doing your cardio on a machine (or at least it helps). You can take this same concept and apply it to any type of cardio machine you have—a treadmill, stationary bike, elliptical trainer, or rowing machine. If you don't have a piece of cardio equipment, no worries. All you need is a four-foot space in front of your TV and you can run in place, do jumping jacks, or simply march it out as you watch your favorite shows or movies. Basically, it's all just about getting off the couch and getting active.

➤ Cool Tip

If your kids like video games, make sure they get interactive video games like those for Wii, and choose games that you need to stand, engage your body, or move around in order to play. This way your kids will be maximizing their video game experience, and you can join in on the fun too! A great example of this is the game Dance Dance Revolution.

- **Get your pump on:** Many times you may not have time to hit the gym, but with a few simple pieces of equipment at your house, you can get in a great strength-training workout. Simple items like a TRX Suspension Training band, push-up handles, a pull-up bar, or a medicine ball are all examples of how to get a pump on at home. Simply go to your local sporting goods store, visit the gym section, and talk to an associate. For a few hundred dollars, you can be set up with the necessary pieces of equipment to keep your strength training rockin' at home when the gym isn't an option. Plus you can also use this equipment for your family obstacle course nights.

- **Sporting battle royale:** Maybe it's a ping-pong battle, a foosball tournament, a Nerf basketball game, or even a water-gun fight. The point is, it's really easy to turn your home into a sporting battle royale. You simply choose the games you and your family like, evaluate your space, get the equipment, and let the sporting battle begin!

- **Rolling and stretching festivities:** After all of this extra activity, a nice massage and adjustment probably sounds pretty good. The only problem, as busy parents, who has time to get a massage? Maybe occasionally, but your muscles and spine need consistent care to prevent injuries. Injuries and pain are the fastest way to derail any exercise plan. This is why foam rollers are so good for you. Add in some stretching with your roller and you have the best available injury-prevention system (besides proper technique in all your activities). Simply turning part of each night into a ten-minute rolling and stretching festival for you and your family will keep your spine adjusted,

your circulation flowing, and your muscles loose and
flexible.

Your life as a watcher is now a thing of the past. Up until this
point, it was probably what you thought being a parent was about,
and it was difficult to find the time to make your exercise happen.
Well, now you have the tools and know that everywhere you go can
become a gym—it just needs your imagination!

Here's a quick recap and your action items from this chapter. And
remember, these are just your starting points. Take each of these, customize them to you, and continue adding more, 1 percent at a time!

At-Work Adventures

Your ho-hum workdays are over. It's time to bring sixty-second-or-
less adventures to your workplace:

- **Who needs a chair?** Use an exercise ball as your new chair.

- **Climb away:** Multiply your stair climbing by two.

- **Sixty-second bursts:** Bust out a sixty-second strength-
  training workout every hour.

- **Water cooler time:** Fill up your water bottle every hour
  from the water station farthest from your desk.

- **Zen moments:** Bring some calmness to your day by doing a
  stretch and listening to your favorite song.

It's Always Game Time

Steal back big chunks of bonus workout time during your extracurricular and lifestyle activities:

- **You don't need a track to walk:** Leave the chair in the car, wear your sneakers, dress for a workout, and get to it.

- **Playground social hour:** Avoid the bench and have fun at the playground. Tighten your core as you slide, have a swinging competition, or play a game of tag.

- **Looks like a sport to me:** Have your sneakers and a ball, and let your imagination take over. Anything can be turned into a sport.

Turn Your Home into a Fitness Fun House

Start living outside the box and make your home a carnival of exercise:

- **Bounce city:** Jump away on a trampoline. It's the easiest way to smile.

- **Obstacle course Friday:** Whether it's Friday or a different night, turn your house into a fun-filled obstacle course for the family.

- **TV and movie experience:** Forget about the couch and get active while watching your favorite shows and movies.

- **Get your pump on:** In the lack of gym time, just pump out some push-ups and pull-ups at home.

- **Sporting battle royale:** No need for pay-per-view here— the battle royale is now at your house. Just set up for your favorite sporting events and let the competition begin.

- **Rolling and stretching festivities:** Need a massage, but time is tight? Keep your body flexible, your spine adjusted, and your muscles loose with a foam roller and ten minutes of stretching each day.

► **Quick Info and Exercise Support Tip**

As your imagination builds and creativity expands, you will continue pushing your exercise boundaries. Your search for more ideas on how to include your family and maximize your workout time will continue to evolve. For this reason, there's additional fitness support through blogs, webinars, coaching videos, etc. Simply visit *www.WhyKidsMakeYouFat.com/ExerciseAdventures*.

You're probably at the place now where you're feeling this and you know you can do it. You're owning your food, and with the strategies presented in this chapter, your watcher days are a thing of the past. You've been inspired by the success stories, and you see the possibility of what can be achieved with your body and what you can work into your world.

But as a parent, you must know there's a piece of the puzzle we haven't yet discussed. I call it your body's X-factor, because when it's out of balance, your progress will halt, your irritability will skyrocket, and your cravings will become uncontrollable. This sneaky X-factor is, of course, stress. Show me parents who say they aren't stressed (at least a little) and I'll make them prove to me they have children. The reality is, we all know we need to reduce our stress; the real question is, how do we do that with a schedule that never seems to stop? Well, this is exactly what you'll learn in chapter 8. It's time to finally implement realistic and doable stress strategies that will help optimize your results, make you less cranky (which makes the entire family happy), and keep you on plan.

8

I Said No!
Oh Great,
I Gained
Another Pound

As parents, I think we've all had those moments when our stress meter was off the chart. It happened to me when Hunter was four and we were at a department store. I had a meeting I needed to be at in thirty minutes, so I went in the store strong and committed to just getting the two things we needed. What ensued was definitely not the plan.

Hunter saw a stuffed animal he really wanted (adding one more to the hundreds he already had) and as I kept saying no, he kept saying yes. As each minute passed, I felt my stress levels rise higher and higher, doing my best to stay calm with my extremely stubborn four-year-old. After my tenth no, Hunter sat down in the middle of the aisle and began to have a full-blown tantrum. I stood there in disbelief, feeling a bit helpless and embarrassed. After thirty minutes passed and I missed my meeting, I caved in, Hunter got his stuffed animal, and I felt exhausted and a pound heavier from the stress! Definitely not one of my finest parenting moments.

The reality of my story is that it happens to parents all the time. Kids are stress producers, and for some unexplainable reason, they know exactly how to push our buttons. The challenge with that is, stress causes an over-release of cortisol (your stress hormone), which is the main culprit in storing belly fat. I call stress your X-factor because it's the unknown saboteur of your results. Your food and exercise could be spot on, but if your stress meter is off the chart, your results and progress will suffer greatly. For this reason, it's crucial you get your stress in check.

Stress and Your Choices

Now, I get it—we all know we need to have less stress in our lives. This isn't a secret to anyone. I wish I could share some magical potion to help you eliminate your stress, but unfortunately that doesn't exist. So until that magical potion is discovered, we each need to manage our stress the old-fashioned way, through our choices.

Think of your kids—every time they get upset or stressed, most likely it was a choice. They chose to react a particular way. Now think of 99 percent of the time you get stressed—most likely that was a choice as well. That tension in your body when you're stuck in traffic, the frustration you experience when your kids aren't ready on time, the increased heart rate and perspiration when you're running late for a meeting, and the anxiety you feel from your kids' bone-chilling screams (those are so annoying!). Each of these examples is a mini-moment of stress, and when they happen too often, your body shifts into chronic stress mode. The mini-moments I'm talking about are not the big stressors of life, like a death in the family or losing a job or suffering an injury. When the big stressors of life hit, you do the best you can to persevere and push through. The stressors I'm talking about are the everyday stressors like the examples I just shared.

You see, each stress mini-moment triggers your body to over-release cortisol (your stress hormone) and adrenaline (your energy hormone). Stress is your body's defense mechanism, and those two hormones in essence prepare you for battle, whatever that battle may be. Once the stress is alleviated, your body shifts into a relaxed state and your hormone levels return to normal. We all know that stress is a natural part of life and, when kept in check, it's fine. The problem comes from when you have too many of these stress mini-moments and your body can't relax between each stress episode. These frequent stress episodes cause high cortisol levels in your blood that lead to elevated blood sugar levels, triggering increased fat storage. They also suppress your immune system, which makes you more susceptible to getting sick as well as experiencing inflammation and bloating. And finally, high cortisol levels slow down your digestion system and make it difficult to metabolize your food. All these factors lead to increases in your weight, body fat, and inches—which is, of course, the opposite of the direction you want to go.

Based on that information, it's obvious that stress can quickly derail your progress. This is why managing your stress needs to be on your radar and a priority during your 8 Week Run and Thrive phase. This chapter is all about implementing three real-world strategies to minimize your stress, decrease the moments you want to pull the hair out of your head due to kid frustration, and empower you to finally slay the X-factor known as stress. Let's dive into your first strategy, stealing back your sleep.

► **Quick Stress Measuring Note**

Since your stress is based on how you feel, let's put a tangible number to it, just like your number on the scale. Each week evaluate your stress and give it a number value between 1 and 10, 10 being the highest level of stress and 1 being lowest level of stress. Each week see if your stress levels are decreasing. This will provide you a tangible way to stay in touch with your stress and monitor your progress.

Strategy 1: Steal Back Your Sleep

I never really understood the statement "I'll sleep when I'm dead" until Hunter was born. There's nothing that jolts you out of bed faster than a crying baby. Seriously, it's the best alarm clock ever created. You would think the older your kids get, the easier it is to fall back into a solid sleep routine, but unfortunately that's just not the case. I'm constantly reminded of my mom's statement, "Being a parent is a twenty-four-hour-a-day job." The sleep-deprived baby and toddler days are replaced with pre-teen slumber parties, followed by late-night worry fests waiting for your teenager to come home. Abbi and I are in the pre-teen slumber-party phase, and man, they can be just as exhausting as the baby nights. My point is, as a parent your golden sleep days may be a thing of the past, but by understanding your sleep, you can find a way to steal many of those precious lost hours back.

Now, you may be thinking, *How does sleep help manage my stress?* I ask you: Are you more stressed when you're tired? Is your fuse shorter after a poor night's rest? Do you crave more comfort and carb-heavy foods when you're fatigued? I'm assuming the answer is yes to all those questions. Your sleep, or lack of it, has a direct effect on your stress levels and your two stress hormones (cortisol and adrenaline), and by simply implementing three tips, you can drastically improve your overall sleep, which will greatly help you minimize your stress.

TIP 1: THE POWER OF 90

Look at your sleep as your body's battery charger, just like electricity charges your cell phone's battery. Your body's battery charging runs in ninety-minute cycles. Your sleep has four stages. Stages one and two are light sleep, and stages three and four are deep sleep. Light sleep prepares your body for deep sleep, and deep sleep repairs and renews your body (tissue, nerve cells, and glands). Your deep sleep is then followed by REM sleep, which stands for rapid eye movement. While deep sleep refreshes your body, REM sleep refreshes your brain by reorganizing its thoughts and memories, like organizing a file cabinet. Once the ninety-minute cycle ends, it circles back around to stage one, light sleep. The graphic on the following page provides an excellent visual of your sleep cycle.

I know this isn't science class, and I promised to keep this book simple and to the point, but trust me, it's important to understand

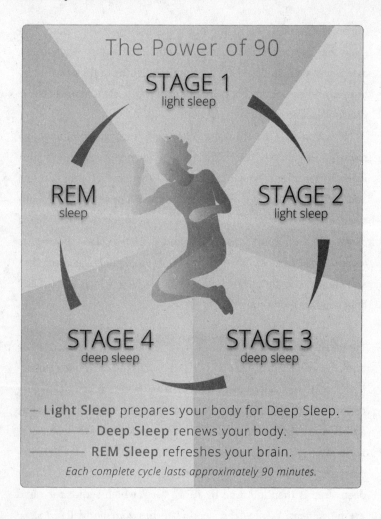

The Power of 90

STAGE 1
light sleep

REM
sleep

STAGE 2
light sleep

STAGE 4
deep sleep

STAGE 3
deep sleep

— **Light Sleep** prepares your body for Deep Sleep. —
———— **Deep Sleep** renews your body. ————
———— **REM Sleep** refreshes your brain. ————
Each complete cycle lasts approximately 90 minutes.

this cycle. Think back to a time when your kid was sleeping deeply and within twenty minutes started to fidget (entering light sleep), when some type of noise was made and she woke up and couldn't fall back to sleep. That's a perfect example of how your sleep cycle works: she just completed a ninety-minute cycle and before she could go through another cycle, the noise woke her up. If the noise had never occurred, she probably would have kept sleeping and repeated another cycle. Now think of a time when you fell asleep with the television on a bit too loud and suddenly woke up. That sudden rousing is simply your body repeating its sleep cycle and reentering light sleep. The noise from the television triggered your sudden awakening and took you out of light sleep mode.

Understanding this is crucial in stealing back your sleep because we've already established and accepted that for parents, endless hours of sleep are not possible, but focusing on ninety-minute sleep increments is possible. For example, if you had a late night and there was potential for a nap the following day, make it a ninety-minute nap. If a nap is out of the question, go to bed ninety minutes earlier. If you're in a massive sleep hole, then get as many ninety-minute cycles in a row as you can. Bottom line, just make sure when you sleep to complete ninety-minute cycles because the quality of your sleep is so much stronger when a full cycle is completed than compared to an interrupted cycle. Also, for longer stretches, make sure to avoid sleeping in loud environments that can abruptly wake you from light sleep and evaporate much-needed sleep minutes. As simple as this tip is, if you can master these sleep cycles, your quality of sleep with be greatly improved.

TIP 2: BREAK THE SNOOZE BUTTON

In college, hitting the snooze button used to be one of my greatest joys. When 6:00 A.M. would roll around, my alarm would go off, I would hit snooze, and for the next thirty minutes, I felt like I was stealing time and sleep. Then I learned about the sleep cycles, and my dreams were shattered. Yes, this tip is true, as hard as it might be—it's time we all break our snooze buttons. The reality is that every second of sleep after you hit the snooze button is useless sleep for your body and mind. Post–snooze button sleep is only light sleep, and as you just learned, light sleep doesn't provide the much-needed deep sleep and REM sleep your body and mind need. By not using your snooze button, you will maximize every second of quality sleep until it's time to wake up. So ditch your snooze button and immediately start stealing back sleep.

TIP 3: GET YOUR DOWNTIME

I remember the baby days of Hunter. Each night we would do our best to get him ready for sleep—a nice soothing bath, relaxing music, comfy pajamas, and we'd cap it off by reading a bedtime story. The nights we followed that pattern, Hunter seemed to sleep so well, and the nights we didn't follow that routine, let's just say Abbi and I paid the price.

It's funny how as adults we forget that we have the same anatomy and physiology as when we were kids. We're just bigger versions of ourselves. Along with forgetting that, we also seem to struggle with creating downtime after a busy day. Your body cannot push all day and then just switch off the adrenaline and pass out. Just as Hunter slept better with his downtime ritual, you will sleep better with one of your own. My suggestion is to find three things that relax you and work them into your bedtime routine. A few examples could be taking a bath, reading a book, listening to music, stretching, surfing the web, or watching television or a movie—basically anything that helps you chill and unwind. Getting your downtime will help you relax, make you fall asleep faster, and improve your quality of sleep—all great perks to stealing back your sleep.

> ► Quick Alcohol Sleep Note

Many times people think alcohol helps them sleep, but that's not the case. Alcohol may help you decompress and enter light sleep, but any benefit stops there. Alcohol actually works against your quality of sleep by disrupting the consistent flow of light sleep to deep sleep to REM sleep. So that glass of wine, bottle of beer, or shot of hard liquor is definitely not your sleep friend. If you're in the Thrive phase and want to occasionally drink, simply try to have your last drink three hours before bed, and the less you drink the better your quality of sleep will be.

Strategy 2: Progress over Perfection

The definition of *perfection* is "the condition, state, or quality of being free or as free as possible from all flaws or defects." Wow, just the idea of that raises my stress levels. For years I chased the concept of perfection. When I struggled with my speech, I wanted to learn how to speak perfectly. As a soccer player, I wanted to play perfectly, and as a fitness model, I wanted to achieve the perfect body. My obsessiveness to be perfect nearly cost me my mind. We all have a breaking point, and when we continually put pressure on ourselves to be perfect we'll eventually crack.

As a kid, teenager, and young adult, every moment I thought I was close to the idea of perfection, the pressure would boil over, my anxiety would overwhelm me, and an avalanche would fall. My worst avalanche happened in my early twenties when I was the most obsessed with making my body perfect. I was spending hours in the gym, eating super clean, and analyzing every inch of my body. When I wasn't working out, I lived in fear of losing the progress I had achieved. When I wanted to eat an off-plan meal, I panicked that every ounce of fat I burned would come back, and when I spent time with Abbi, my mind was in a different place thinking about my next workout, the supplements I needed, or my food. As we all know, there is only one outcome for this type of obsessiveness—a complete crash and burn—and in my case, I fell into a deep depression. My mythological drive for perfection temporarily broke me.

I was in a tough place, but two things that the smartest person I know in this world—my wife, Abbi—shared with me pulled me out of my depression. First, she reminded me that perfection was only a myth and that I would never speak perfectly, play soccer perfectly, have the perfect body, or basically do anything perfectly because it's an unattainable goal and chasing an unattainable goal is what was causing my obsession. Abbi then kindly reminded me of the motto I've lived since I was seven years old: 1 percent progress. Abbi's wisdom pulled me out of that dark place, and an enhanced motto was born: progress over perfection.

It's a concept that sounds great on paper and seems so simple. It's also one of the most difficult things to live by. Think of the dieting industry—more people are focused on their health than ever before, and there is more available information than ever before, yet our health as a society continues to regress. Why is that? Part of it is due to information overload, which is exactly why I wrote this book to provide information with guidance. And the other reason is because the popular concept of dieting is all about being perfect.

The idea of being perfect is exactly what Heather Hartman wanted every time she dieted. It was her moment to be perfect, drop her clothing sizes, and finally shed the pounds that had haunted her for so many years. As a working mom, her stress was always high, and every time she would lose some weight, the pressures of life would push back, shatter her idea of perfection, and trigger a

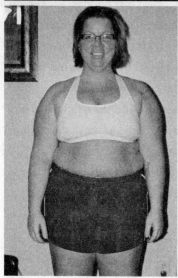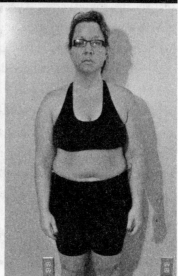

Heather Hartman

2 years before   before 8 weeks

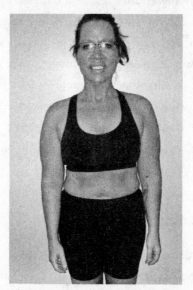

after 8 weeks

bout of emotional eating to counter her stress. It was at this point that Heather found herself at her heaviest, 287 pounds. She couldn't believe that all her past diets and her focus on perfection had left her heavier and unhappier with her body than she had ever been.

At that moment Heather decided it was time for a mind-set shift. Heather went from chasing perfection and stress eating to focusing on daily progress. This new mind-set immediately relieved the pressure she had felt with every diet, and if she had a bad day with her food, she would simply let it go and get right back on track. Now, this wasn't an easy transition for Heather, but each day she chipped away and started making progress, and over a two-year period, Heather dropped fifty-five pounds. This is when I met Heather, and with her new mind-set, she was ready to ramp up her effort and make her 8 Week Run. And boy, did she. In eight weeks, Heather lost thirty pounds, twenty inches, and four sizes. And after seven months of Thriving, Heather lost an additional twenty-one pounds, twelve inches, and two more sizes. To date, Heather has lost a total of 106 pounds, and most important, she has a new motto that will ensure her results keep on coming: progress over perfection.

Implementing this strategy of progress over perfection will be a huge step in eliminating all the unnecessary pressure and stress that losing weight and reaching for your perfect body create. It's not a complex concept; it's simply a mind-set shift on how you look at things as you live your plan.

Strategy 3: Control—Let It Go

Just as perfection is a myth, I consider *control* a deadly seven-letter word. For parents, control is our safe haven. It's an imaginary land we all pretend we live in, and that land of control is definitely a powerful stress-producing machine. I get it, and I'm guilty of it as well. The idea of the unknown is not the easiest thing to accept, especially with our kids.

See, before kids, we had a sense of control over our actions and choices, but once we became parents, that calm sense of control flew right out the window. I remember my most vivid memory of this. Hunter was two years old, and I wanted him to tie his shoes and he didn't want to. We went back and forth, and I finally yelled, "Hunter, tie your shoes!" (of course wanting to add some expletives to that statement).

He asked, "Why?"

I replied, "Because I said so."

He then stared me down, looked me right in the eyes, and said, "You're not the boss of me!"

I was in shock, frustrated, and mad, which are all excellent emotional cortisol producers. It was that moment when I realized Abbi's and my life had changed forever. The control we once imagined we had was gone.

But lack of control goes deeper than wanting our kids to do what we want them to do, when we want them to do it. As I shared in the food frenzy chapter, simply dealing with your kid getting sick, or having a sport tournament, or experiencing a tough day at school can throw a wrench in your entire schedule, and any ounce of control you thought you had is immediately gone.

What I love about Abbi is that control is barely in her DNA, and it's helped me a ton. Abbi's always been a free spirit, moving with the breeze, easily letting things roll off her shoulder, and just not taking life so seriously. As you can guess, Abbi's definitely not a type-A personality. She constantly asks me, "Mark, seriously, does it really matter?" At first I was so annoyed by that question. *What is she thinking? Of course it matters,* I'd think, not even really knowing what "it" was.

But what I've realized is, the more I try to control things, the more stress and pressure I put on myself. That's why this strategy is also a simple mind-set shift like progress over perfection. Control is not a tangible thing—it's a thought, a feeling, and a desire that you choose to focus on or not. Now, don't get me wrong. I still like the idea that I'm in control at times, but I also needed to accept the hard truth that if I wanted to minimize my stress, I needed to simply let a lot of my idea of control go.

So this is my advice to you: If your personality is more like Abbi's, this isn't a big deal for you, but if you're more like me and have been called a control freak or type-A (such endearing terms), try this suggestion the next time you enter control land. Simply ask yourself, "Seriously, does it really matter?" That simple question lets you take a step back and reflect for a moment. If it does matter, then go for it, but I think that you'll slowly and surely realize, just like I did, that most things you're attempting to control do not really matter. This adjustment will drastically help you reduce your stress.

Control is something my dear friend Javier Solis had to let go of as well. I was speaking at an event, and Javi came up to me seeming super stressed and unhappy. We sat down, and he started sharing how he was struggling to make everything work with the pressures of life. He hated that his health wasn't great and that he was exhausted after work. He was working a lot of hours, and the unhealthier he became, the more he felt a lack of control with his food, exercise, and quality time with his family. He wanted to be a better husband to his wife, Pavela, and father to their three kids. Javi was tired of trying to control each element of his life and knew that if he could get his health back in check, his mood, stress, and energy

Javier Solis

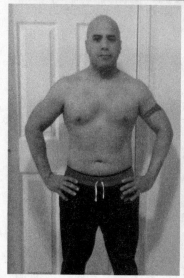
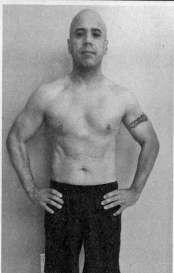

before   after 8 weeks

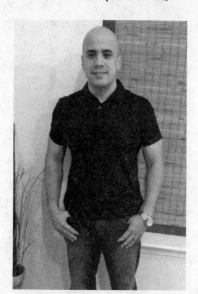

beyond 8 weeks

Pavela Solis

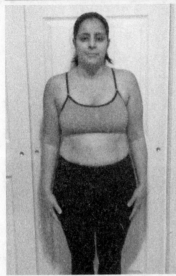

before

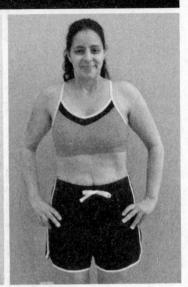

after 8 weeks

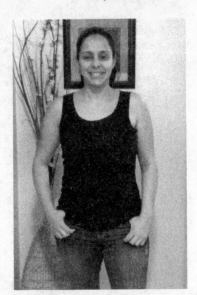

beyond 8 weeks

would all improve. Javi also shared that Pavela was struggling with stress and needed to find ways to manage it better. Javier and Pavela made their 8 Week Run together and rocked their plan. Javier lost twenty-three pounds, eighteen inches, and two pants sizes in eight weeks and has lost an additional eight pounds, four inches, and one pants size in his Thrive phase. Pavela lost twenty-four pounds, twenty-three inches, and two sizes in eight weeks and an additional twelve pounds, eight inches, and one pants size during her Thrive phase.

But the success of Javier and Pavela goes beyond their external results. Both of their stress levels greatly decreased, and Javier achieved his goal, becoming the dad and husband he wanted to be.

As we know, there is no magical potion for eliminating stress. Your real solution is choosing how you react to your stressors. Here's a quick recap and action items from this chapter to minimize your stress and optimize your results.

Rate Your Stress 1 through 10

Each week evaluate your stress. Just like you weigh yourself and measure your inches, measure your stress, 10 being the highest level of stress and 1 being the lowest level of stress. Each week see if your stress levels are decreasing. This provides you with a tangible way to monitor your stress levels.

Steal Back Your Sleep

- **The power of 90:** You now know the science of your sleep and its stages. Make sure to keep your sleep in ninety-minute cycles to maximize each stage of sleep and REM.

- **Break your snooze button:** Ditch the snooze button and sleep deeply till it's time to wake up. Every second of post–snooze button sleep is useless.

- **Get your downtime:** Remember, you sleep better with downtime, just like your kids do, so find three relaxing things and start decompressing before bed. Also remember, alcohol is not your bedtime friend.

Progress over Perfection

- **Perfection is a myth:** Chasing a perfect body will always leave you empty-handed and frustrated. Understand the concept of perfection doesn't exist.

- **1% progress:** This is the theme of the entire book, daily 1 percent progress.

- **If you fall off, just get back on:** We all fall off plan. If you fall off, don't stress—just get right back on.

Control—Let It Go

- **Control is an imaginary land:** We live there, but it's not tangible. It's a thought, a feeling, and a desire that we choose to focus on or not.

- **Ask yourself, "Seriously, does it really matter?"** This simple question keeps you in check and helps you evaluate if trying to control a situation is important or a waste of time, energy, and stress.

Congratulations, you're now at your golden moment. The moment you complete what you started. The moment you draw your line in the sand. The moment you stay consistent and in rhythm. The moment you finish strong. Your first eight chapters provided you with the tools to win with your plan and take your body and health to the next level. Now it's time to cross the finish line. That's what chapter 9 is all about, providing you with the inspiration and motivation to forever own your health, live your plan fully, and sprint full speed through the finish line. Final chapter, here we come.

9

Crossing the Finish Line

My friend Kelli Bonomo told me for years that she wanted to get back in shape and lose weight. She knew what to do, but for some reason, she just wasn't doing it. Kelli's struggles were similar to what most parents deal with—basically, a sheer lack of time. She's a mom and a wife and she works, so regardless of how hard she tried, she couldn't find the time to make her health happen. In her pre-kid days, she could make herself a priority. She could create the time she needed for herself, but not now—she didn't have that same freedom anymore. So she was left frustrated and fed up, living a semi-happy life—happy of course with her kids and husband, Mike, but completely discouraged and depressed about her own body and weight. She hit a point where she was close to just settling and accepting the fact that this might be her new body and that her past days of being happy and satisfied with her health were no longer a reality.

Unfortunately, this is the conclusion many parents end up moving toward. They get tired of the fight and the constant struggle of trying to balance everything, and for a moment it feels easier and lessens the pressure to begin thinking this is how it's supposed to be. I've been coaching clients including parents since 1995, and I understand how hard it is to make your health work. It's why I wrote this book.

I went to Kelli and shared with her that I got that she knew what to do, but it was time she stop focusing on what had worked for her in the past and begin focusing on what can work now, as a parent, when her time isn't always hers. I coached Kelli through her 8 Week Run, and she lost thirty pounds, eleven inches, and four sizes and finally found the body, health, and confidence that had left her for so many years.

But what makes Kelli's story even more powerful is that her success inspired her teenage daughter, Kaytlyn Harsha, to know that she didn't have to starve herself in order to have the body she wanted. Kelli's leading by example showed Kaytlyn what was possible and motivated her to take action, dropping thirty-five pounds and four dress sizes in eight weeks. Kaytlyn's transformation illustrates what this book is truly about—educating fellow parents like Kelli on how to permanently achieve their health goals so they can show their families how to do the same. This is how we stop the dieting madness and start living the quality of life we deserve. Which leads me to my favorite picture in this book. Check out Kaytlyn's joy and newfound confidence: just seeing her picture makes you want to smile.

The successes of Kelli, Kaytlyn, and every other person in this book can be your success. All they did was live the plan and take

Kelli Bonomo

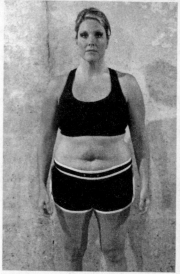

before

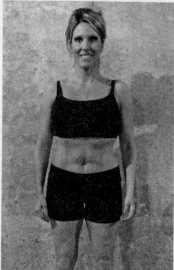

after 8 weeks

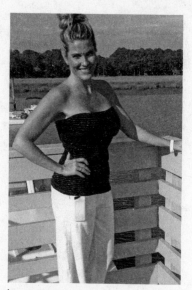

beyond 8 weeks

Kaytlyn Harsha

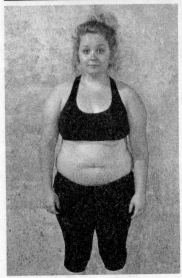

before

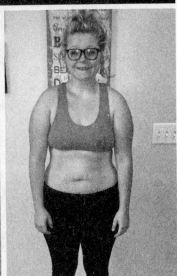

after 8 weeks

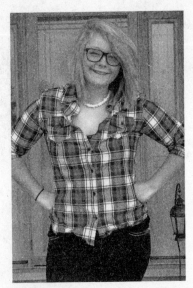

beyond 8 weeks

the coaching you've learned in this book. The information, plug-and-play plans, and strategies are your core pieces to unlocking your body's full potential and taking your health to the next level. The big question now is, how can you cross the finish line like the champion you are?

Think back to everything you've started in your life. Most likely you started strong, motivated, and on fire. Now think back to everything you've finished strong in your life. Most likely you've started more things than you've finished—we all have! The question you need to ask yourself is, why? What makes you quit something or continue moving forward? What causes you to stop short of the finish line compared to bursting through it? What makes you lose hope in what can be or still see the light of possibility? These are great questions to ask yourself, and there are no right or wrong answers.

What I know is that making your health happen is not the easiest thing. It takes hard work, dedication, and the ability to push through those tough moments. There are costs to everything in life, and my simple litmus test is to ask yourself this question: Is the juice worth the squeeze? If you've made fresh-squeezed juice, then you know how time consuming and energy draining that can be compared to the simplicity of just buying some juice in a carton. Sometimes it's worth squeezing it yourself, and sometimes it's not.

I invite you to ask yourself that same question about your health. There are no easy rides, and if you want to truly reprogram your metabolism and permanently lose weight, then you will—you just have to make sure the juice is worth the squeeze and be ready to do the work. Here are the three concepts that will help you cross the finish line like a champion and ensure the juice is worth the squeeze!

Make Yourself a Priority

Wow, this is a tough one for us parents. We're trained that being selfish is a bad thing. Of course, sometimes it can be, but many times you need to make a stand for your health and draw your line in the sand. If doing that is defined as being a little selfish, then you need to start being a little selfish for your 8 Week Run and beyond. If all you do is give of yourself and take nothing back, then your health will always come second and your goals will never be achieved.

Making yourself a priority simply means setting boundaries that keep you on track with enough flexibility that lets you be the parent you need to be. In this book you've learned so many ways to make your food and exercise realistically work that now you simply need to find the concepts and strategies that work best for you, live the plan, and set your boundaries. Teach your family that you are a priority and they should join you in this journey so you all live your health together.

Stay in Rhythm

In life you're either in rhythm or you're in a rut. A rhythm creates consistency, and a rut leads to boredom, which will eventually make you fall off plan. In your pre-kid days, it was probably easier to stay in rhythm and avoid a rut because you had less responsibility and more time. As parents we fight the daily time crunch that leads to more hectic days. That chaos can quickly pull us out of rhythm, but in addition, because time is harder to find, we tend to become creatures of habit and stop experimenting with new foods or finding new workouts. Eventually boredom sets in, and we fall out of rhythm and off plan.

Staying in rhythm is more of a mind-set to always realize that you're a moment away from losing consistency and you must maintain awareness and continue to diversify your foods and exercise to prevent the dreaded rut.

Finish Strong and Lead by Example

You're tired, you've pushed, and you're almost on empty. That's the feeling you get when you push yourself to the limit. Finishing strong is about challenging yourself and taking your body and mind to a place it hasn't seen or been before.

In the movie *Superman Returns,* Superman lifts an island made of kryptonite and launches it into space, to save the world. As he releases the island, he falls back to Earth, completely exhausted. I love that visual of Superman giving everything he had—all of his heart, strength, and dedication—to a cause that was worth fighting for. That visual of Superman reminds me of Shannon Webber.

The Webber family started their 8 Week Run as one powerful unit, a family of seven—Shannon, Scott, and their five kids. Shannon had grown up a chronic dieter, struggling to manage her weight and being raised by her grandparents with food as comfort and a reward. She then passed that philosophy on to her children—it was all she knew. When her children started having weight issues and struggles with their body confidence, she knew it was time to make a stand for herself and for them. Just like Superman, or Superwoman in Shannon's case, she gave everything. Shannon knew this was something worth fighting for. The emotional weight challenges and insecurities she lived with were never supposed to be passed down to her kids. Those were her battles, not theirs. She needed to make sure her kids wouldn't suffer as she had for so many years. Shannon led the charge, and her action of leading by example

Shannon Webber

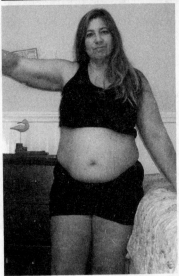

before

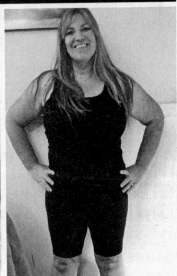

after 8 weeks

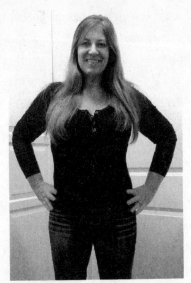

beyond 8 weeks

became the inspiration and motivation for her family on their 8 Week Run. Eight weeks later, Shannon had lost thirty pounds and thirty inches and her family had dropped a combined 146 pounds and 135 inches. Fast-forward through eight months of Thriving, and Shannon has now lost a total of sixty-two pounds and forty-six inches, and the Webber family is down by a total of 227 pounds and 182 inches! That's what I call finishing strong!

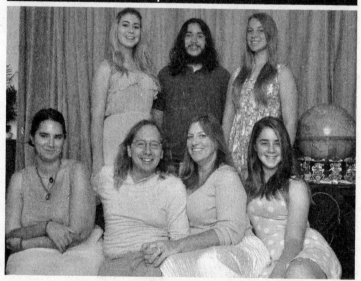

The Webber Family

down 227 pounds and 182 inches in 10 months

Crossing the finish line is about making yourself a priority, staying in rhythm, finishing strong, and leading by example. It's now time for our journey together with this book to come to a close, but before you move on, using the tools and rocking your plan on your own and with our support community, I want to leave you with some final thoughts.

Abbi and I always talk about living our dream. To us that means living the fullest, happiest, and most powerful life we can. In our life together, through every step we've taken in pursuit of our goals, our health has been the main factor in determining our happiness. In essence our health is the "why" behind how we live and so much more than numbers on a scale. Our health provides us with the energy to have a conversation with one another at the end of a long, tiring day, or to play a game of catch or a board game with Hunter instead of zoning out in front of the TV, or to take on the weekend and create incredible family adventures like bike riding in the mountains, hitting an amusement park, or simply going for a family walk with our dogs. Bottom line, when you strip it all down, making our health a priority gives us the ability to feel free, alive, and full of energy again, just like when we were kids.

That's what I love about kids. They are incredible in the way they see the world, the way they take on the world, and the way they live fully engaged in every moment. But as parents we must remember we were also once kids and to not lose ourselves and the importance of our own health as we experience the unbelievable joy of being a parent. Abbi and I will once again be fully tested on this. We're excited to share that after four years of trying and Abbi suffering a couple of miscarriages, the Macdonald family is expanding with our baby girl, named Hope. And this time around, we are taking on the chaos of being parents fully prepared and ready to win—no scale increases or expanding waistlines are in our future! It's funny to think that Abbi and I will be sixty years old when Hope is eighteen. That's crazy! But you better believe our "why" just got even stronger. We want to live life with Hope and Hunter to the fullest, and the only way that's possible is by always making our health a priority and a permanent focus in our lives.

So that leads me to ask, what does living your dream mean to you? As you take on the world, what type of parent and person do you want to be? What example do you want to set for your kids? Because here's what I know: without your health, you cannot be the person you dream of being or the parent you want to be.

My message to you is this: You can have it all. You can be your best. You can have your health and be the parent, spouse, and person you dream of being. You simply have to make the choice that your time is now, your moment is here.

There are many things you cannot control in this world. The one thing you can is how you choose to take care of yourself. It all begins with a choice, and remember: your transformation always starts with *you*!

> ➤ **Support Note Reminder**
>
> As you live your plan it's important to remember that you have an entire community living the Detox, Ignite, and Thrive phases right by your side. For new food or recipe ideas, creative exercise plans, additional motivation, or simply to have your questions answered, plug into your support community at *www.WhyKidsMakeYouFat.com/Community*. You aren't walking this journey alone; we are all walking it together!

Supplement Reference Section

Your 8 Week Run is all about taking your body and health to the next level. You can accomplish this by simply following the food, exercise, and water recommendations in your Detox, Ignite, and Thrive phases as well as utilizing the recipes and coaching content throughout the book.

If you want to turbocharge your plan and maximize your results, here's a consolidated list of recommended, high-quality, natural supplements to fill in your meal and nutrition gaps. These recommendations are based on what research supports as well as what I and our Venice Nutrition practices have seen work best for all who live the plan.

You can get these recommended products at your local vitamin store, health facility, online, or directly from the manufacturer. In addition, I helped develop a product line specifically to work hand in hand with the Detox, Ignite, and Thrive phases and deliver optimal results. The product line is called Zen and is manufactured by Jeunesse.

This reference section is presented in four parts, and some of the content has already been previously shared in the book. The reference section is designed to provide you a snapshot of each supplement and when it fits into your plan. Look at this as your supplement cheat sheet. Here are the four parts:

Part 1: Protein Powders and Meal Replacements (bars and ready-to-drink shakes for your Detox, Ignite, and Thrive phases)

Part 2: Detox Phase Supplementation

Part 3: Ignite Phase Supplementation

Part 4: Thrive Phase Supplementation

➤ **Important Note:**
Four Points to Be Clear on Before You Read This Reference Section

- If you currently have a medical challenge, are pregnant or nursing, or are taking medication prescribed by a physician, consult with your doctor before taking any supplements recommended in this book.

- Protein powders, bars, and ready-to-drink shakes are considered food and are different than the supplements recommended for the Detox, Ignite, and Thrive phases. Look at these protein recommendations as part of your meal plan. You can of course eat whole food every meal if you prefer.

- Review your meal plans for each phase to know when and what dosage/serving you should be using for each phase.

- If you're currently taking vitamins, minerals, or antioxidants, please continue with your current routine.

If any product that you're taking has calories from protein, fat, or carbohydrates, please make sure to account for that in your meal plan.

Part 1: Protein Powders and Meal Replacements

Protein Powders

Protein powders contain mainly protein and usually a small amount of carbs and fat. Please make sure to carefully read the nutrition label and serving size. Each powder makes for a differently flavored shake, so choose the flavor you prefer. Here's your protein powder litmus test to ensure you choose a quality protein powder:

- The powder needs at least 20 grams of protein per serving.

- There must be more protein in the powder than carbs and fat.

- The protein source needs to be either whey (hydrolyzed, isolate, or concentrate), micellar casein, egg white, or plant based and not contain soy protein. It can have trace amounts of soy in the form of soy lecithin, which has very little soy and is a binder in shakes.

- The powder needs to be gluten-free.

- The powder needs to be low in sugar and use a natural sweetener (like stevia). There are a few good protein powders that use small amounts of sucralose (fake sugar). If sucralose causes you to experience digestive challenges, avoid it.

The following recommended brands of protein shakes are approved Detox, Ignite, and Thrive phases and can be found at your local supplement store, health facility, or online:

- Zen Fuze shakes, made by Jeunesse with micellar casein and whey, all-natural ingredients and flavored with stevia

- Power Crunch Proto Whey powder, with hydrolyzed whey, made by BNRG

- Egg white protein powder—many quality brands and options

- Warrior Blend plant-based powder, made by Sunwarrior

- Vega One Nutritional Shake, plant-based powder, made by Vega

Protein Bars and Ready-to-Drink Shakes

These are much more processed than protein powder (and the shakes we make from it), so protein bars and ready-to-drink shakes (RTD) are really just for emergencies. Avoid them during your Detox phase and ideally limit yourself to just one bar or ready-to-drink shake once per day during your Ignite and Thrive phases. Here's your litmus test for choosing a protein bar or RTD. It's similar to the guidelines I shared about protein powders. Each bar and RTD has different flavors, so choose the flavor you prefer.

- The protein in the bar or RTD needs to be within a five gram range of the total carbs. For example, if the food label shows twenty grams of carbohydrates, you can eat a bar that has anywhere between fifteen and twenty-five grams of protein. Staying within this five gram range ensures the bar or RTD will be correctly balanced. If the bar has more than five grams more carbs than protein, do not eat it; it will most likely spike your blood sugar.

- The protein source needs to be either whey (hydrolyzed, isolate, or concentrate), micellar casein, egg white, or plant based and must not contain soy protein. It can have trace amounts of soy in the form of soy lecithin, which has very little soy and is a binder in most protein products.

- The bar or RTD needs to be gluten-free.

- The bar needs to be low in sugar, preferably high in fiber, and use a natural sweetener (like stevia). Most RTDs use small amounts of sucralose (fake sugar). If sucralose causes you to experience digestive challenges, avoid it.

Recommended brands of protein bars that pass this litmus test are:

- **Power Crunch:** made by BNRG, preferably choose gluten-free options

- **Quest:** made by Quest, gluten-free

- **Rise Protein Bar:** made by Rise, gluten-free

Recommended brands of RTDs that pass the litmus test are:

- **Power Crunch:** made by BNRG

- **Muscle Milk:** made by CytoSport

Part 2: Detox Phase Supplementation

The following supplements and dosages are designed to clean out your liver, kidneys, and colon. There are cleansing supplements and two bowel regulatory supplements.

I helped develop Zen Prime Cleanse, which contains all the recommended cleansing supplements and is designed specifically for the Detox phase. You can purchase Zen Prime or the individual cleansing ingredients from your local supplement store, health facility, or online.

Detox Cleanse Supplements

- **Zen Prime Cleanse:** made by Jeunesse, contains all recommended ingredients to cleanse your liver, kidneys, and colon. Take two tablets per day during your Detox phase.

- **Milk thistle (liver cleanse):** 500 mg (100 mg of silybum marianum) once a day during your Detox phase

- **Cranberry extract (kidney cleanse):** 500 mg once a day during your Detox phase

- **Dandelion Root (diuretic and colon):** 1500 mg once a day

- **Digestive Enzyme Blend (digestive and colon):** 250–300 mg once a day

Bowel Regularity and Additional Gentle Detox Tea

If you struggle with constipation or would like some extra colon cleansing for increased regularity, here is one supplement and a tea (available online, at health food stores, and at most grocery stores) that will help. They can also be taken during your Ignite and Thrive phases.

- **Psyllium husk (fiber—soluble and insoluble):** 5 g (in fiber or capsule) twice a day

- **EveryDay Detox Tea, made by Traditional Medicinals:** one tea bag per day

Part 3: Ignite Phase Supplementation

The following supplements are designed to burn body fat, restore your intestinal health, and increase the health of your heart, skin, hair, and nails. For the Ignite phase, I helped develop Zen Shape, a metabolism booster (fat burner), and the Zen Fuze shakes, created with five different strains of probiotics; both products are made by Jeunesse.

You can purchase the Zen Ignite products, or you can individually purchase the ingredients from your local supplement store, health facility, or online. Just make sure the quality of any product you take is good and worth the cost.

Metabolism-Boosting Supplements (Fat Burners)

- **Zen Shape:** made by Jeunesse, contains green tea, chromium polynicotinate. Take two capsules, twice a day, 30 minutes before a meal, during your Ignite phase

If you are not using Zen Shape, then take both the following metabolism-boosting ingredients during your Ignite phase:

- **Green tea (50% caffeine):** 250 mg twice a day, 30 minutes before a meal, during your Ignite phase

- **Chromium polynicotinate:** 200 mcg twice a day, 30 minutes before a meal, during your Ignite phase

➤ **Important Metabolism-Boosting Supplement Note**

If your goal is to burn additional fat after your Ignite phase, stop taking the metabolism boosters for two weeks, and then repeat usage for eight weeks. Make sure to cycle eight weeks on, two weeks off, so your body doesn't get used to the thermogenic (fat-burning) effect.

Probiotics—For Your Ignite and Thrive Phases

- **Zen Fuze Shake:** made by Jeunesse, a five-strain probiotic blend that contains over 4 billion live bacteria. Take one packet, once a day, during your Ignite and Thrive phases

If you are not using Zen Fuze Shake for your probiotics, then take one of the following supplements:

- **Align:** made by Procter & Gamble, an over-the-counter probiotic available at pharmacies. Take one capsule per day during your Ignite and Thrive phases

- **Acidophilus:** available at all health food stores, an over-the-counter live bacteria strain. Read the label for recommended daily dosage during your Ignite and Thrive phases

Omega-3 Fatty Acids—For Your Ignite and Thrive Phases

To get your necessary omega-3 fatty acids, you can use fish oil, or if you're plant based, choose flax or hemp oil or seeds. If you choose fish oil, make sure it's pharmaceutical grade.

Take *one* of the following supplements, depending on if you are plant based or not:

- **Pharmaceutical-grade fish oil:** 3,000 mg per day

- **Flax or hemp seed or oil (plant based):** 3,000 mg per day

Part 4: Thrive Phase Supplementation

Your Detox and Ignite phases have two types of supplements: result-specific supplements and everyday supplements. The result-specific supplements are primarily for that particular phase, while the everyday supplements are designed for that phase as well as your Thrive phase.

Result-Specific Supplements

- **Detox cleanse supplements:** Only use these during the Detox phase or when you reboot your plan.

- **Metabolism boosters (fat burners) and muscle protectors (amino acids):** These supplements can be cycled eight weeks on, two weeks off.

Everyday Supplements

- Protein shakes

- Protein bars and RTDs (Ignite and Thrive phases only, max one per day)

- Fiber (psyllium husk)

- EveryDay Detox Tea

- Probiotics

- Omega-3s

Acknowledgments

This book holds a very special place in my heart, and it's been an incredible adventure living it and writing it. My goal was simple: to provide real solutions for every parent wanting to make his or her health happen. Our life experiences become our greatest teaching moments, and fortunately they become our wisdom. Our wisdom also comes from the special people in our lives. Many of these people have been instrumental in helping me create this book, and I would like to give them many thanks, massive hugs, and the credit they've earned and deserve. This book would not have become what it is without their help.

My wife, Abbi—You are my partner in crime and the most amazing person in this world. Every step I take, you're there by my side. Every hug I need, you're there to give it. Every conversation I must share, you're there to listen. For the past twenty-one years, you've provided me every ounce of strength, courage, and love that I needed. Words will never give justice to my love and utter appreciation for you, so I'll wrap up simply—I love you.

My son, Hunter—*Heart, passion,* and *courage* are the three words that come to mind when I think of you. Your heart flows with such a pure love for life and people. Your passion drives you to explore every adventure. Your courage empowers you to push the boundaries and reach for the extraordinary. You are my greatest teacher, son. I'm so proud of you, and it's an honor to be your dad.

My baby girl, Hope—Hope, such an incredible name for you and so true to the path we've walked to bring you into this world. Your mom, brother, and I have waited so long for you. I know you'll be Daddy's little girl and will take on life full throttle, just like your mom and brother. I love you, baby girl.

Mom and Dad—As I wrote this book as well as *Body Confidence,* I chuckled about how ingrained you both are in everything I do. There are sprinkles of you, Mom and Dad, in every chapter I write, memories that inspire me to share real life lessons that you taught me. Your unconditional love and support mean the world to me and have allowed me to reach for the stars and become the man I wanted to be. You are both simply the best.

My sisters—Laurie and Chris, the older I get, the more I cherish you both. Laurie, your ability to do everything is astonishing and motivating. You are truly a supermom! Chris, I love that we are tighter than ever. Always remember, the world is yours.

Nancy Hancock—*Visionary* is my word for you. A simple thirty-minute conversation with you inspires me to create something better than I ever thought I could. Your nuggets of wisdom are truly what make you the greatest editor. You've always believed in me and have helped me write the books I've wanted to write without compromise. We are friends and family for life. Love you, NH.

Michael Broussard, Greg Ray, and Michelle Lemons-Poscente (Team ISB)—The amazing three amigos. Michael, you're incredible. As my book agent, you always support my vision, my mission, and me. I love our partnership, what we've accomplished together, and most importantly, our friendship. Greg and Michelle, you've both been instrumental to me these past five years, and the opportunities you introduced to me have been life changing. I want to thank the three of you for your continued belief in me, and I'm excited about the next adventures we will walk together. Family for life, my friends. I will forever appreciate you for helping me live my dreams.

HarperCollins Publishing and Gideon Weil—*Trust, patience,* and *quality* are the three words that come to mind when I think of Team HarperOne. This is our second book together, and I love the team. I love your commitment to creating a powerful book that can lead significant change. I also want to share a special thanks to Gideon Weil—from one dad to another, thank you for your much-appreciated help, valuable insight, and focus on making this book great. Lisa Zuniga—thanks for your dedication, efficiency, and fun spirit; you're such an awesome production editor. And Ali McCart—so appreciate your suggestions and incredible copyediting skills. Ralph Fowler—greatly appreciate your incredible work in designing the book and helping make the content easy to read and alive.

Vaughan Risher—Thank you for always taking the picture I have in my head and turning it into a visual masterpiece. Your skills are special, V, and you were a big part in bringing life to this book with your graphics. Our journey together only gets stronger.

Valerie Cogswell—Chef Valerie, definitely the greatest chef I know. Your ability to make clean and healthy food burst with flavor is second to none. I so appreciate all you did for this book, sharing your delicious blood sugar–balancing recipes and leading all our fellow recipe contributors. You're one of a kind, Val, and family for life.

8 Week Run and Thrive success stories—Thank you Ivette, Gina, Jose, Michelle, Scott, Tracey, Leyla, Sherry, Kelly, Mark, JJ, Heather, Javier, Pavela, Kelli, Kaytlyn, Shannon, and the entire Webber family for inspiring us all and showing what is truly possible with your health. Each of your stories is powerful, motivating, and part of what makes this book complete. My love to you all.

8 Week Run and Thrive Recipe contributors—Thank you, Chef Valerie, Cashawn McTeer Kirbas, Cassandra Ballon Christie, Kate Flatt, Daniel Miller (aka "Plant-Based Man"), Shannon Davis, Dawn McGee, Jennifer Fleischer, Paula Lippert, and Rosie Plimpton for showing every reader that they too can make clean and healthy food yummy. As each recipe is made, you'll know you've helped someone prevent boredom and stay on plan. Much appreciation, recipe gurus!

Team HLN and CNN—Incredible gratitude for our partnership and the amazing opportunity to deliver a message of health consistently on national media. Many thanks and massive hugs to the entire HLN and CNN team for all we do together. Huge appreciation and love to my buddies Don Lemon, Andreas Preuss, Christi Paul, Randi Kaye, Victor Blackwell, and Nadia Bilchik for our great times on CNN. Plus a very special thanks to HLN Now and *The Daily Share* executive producer Jennifer Williams for simply being the best executive producer in the industry as well as a dear friend, and for possessing the leadership to make a difference every day. Also a big thanks to Mike "The Machine" Galanos for his friendship, heart, and passion. You're what every fifty-year-old man should strive for. Plus big hugs to Lynn Berry and Yasmin Vossoughian, for being two incredible anchors who love health. And finally, standing ovation to producers Hanna, Shannon, Stacy, Lynette, and the ladies that do it all, Cameron and Tracey, plus my main man, Dallas, and hats off to Toya and the incredible women in the makeup room.

My Venice Nutrition Partners—What a journey we've walked, and it gets better with every step. My wife Abbi, the operational guru, I love working with you and building something special. Matt Carolan and Dave Jaureguy, the tech gurus and my brothers, thanks for meeting me at Chili's back in the day—now that was a start of something great. Words will never express how much you both mean to me. Donna Lanzillotti Lee, the business guru, your special insight, knowledge, and heart have meant the world and your unwavering passion to make a difference is awe-inspiring. Andrea Neenan, the financial guru, thanks for always being there for Abbi and me. Your love and wisdom are so appreciated and forever cherished. I love each of you so much; together we are making a powerful difference.

Monavie/MYNT team and community—We started our partnership a few years ago, and it has been one of the greatest partnerships of my life. Together we have created a product line that's all natural, high quality, and effective and have helped thousands of people. Much love and thanks to Mauricio, Dallin, Henry, Randy L., Katy, Alex O., Paul M., Austin L., Jim M., Graden, Steve J., Brandon, Tyson, Jeff P., Veronica, James Q., Eric E., Alex G., Bee Jay, Daren, Kristy, Kim P., Ali, Natalie, Wendy W., Kurt, Sandra, Kim and Hailey C., and the entire Monavie/MYNT team for their leadership, hard work, and, most important, friendship. And some special thanks to Mauricio Bellora, Paul Muehlmann, and Austin Larsen for seeing the power and importance of mainstream products and the difference we could make together. To Dallin Larsen for the opportunity and his incredible friendship, and to the entire community of members and leaders for their inspiration and motivation. We are family for life. *Jeunesse/Zen Team and community*—It's a rarity in life when two visions can seamlessly align and passions unite to make a forever impact in the world. Our partnership is something that can and is creating everlasting change in the world. I want to give massive hugs and thanks to Wendy and Randy Lewis for your special hearts, Scott Lewis for the vision and courage to make a powerful difference, and Rob Dawson for making sure all stays aligned behind the scenes. Plus, a huge shout out to my zen project 8 partner, media personality, and digital specialist Cassiah Jay; I love the work we do together. And finally, a huge appreciation and thank you to the entire Jeunesse leadership team, a few being Mark P., Meredith B., Katy and Derek Holt Larsen, Lucy W., Donna A., and of course everyone in our incredible and inspiring community. You each motivate me to work harder and be better every day.

Katy Holt Larsen—I'm forever grateful for your strength and courage to fight the necessary fights and never back down. Thank you for your friendship and leadership; you and I always talk about how everything in life is a season; well our season is just getting started and is one without an ending!

Alex Ochart and Ryan Brown—The marketing gurus. Ninja, your wisdom is priceless and your vision is incredible. Thank you for helping me see how to make a greater difference while always staying true to me. Ryan, your work ethic and ability to deliver cutting-edge ideas is powerful and amazing.

Venice Nutrition Leadership Team—Nicole, Steve, Bryen, Vaughan, Valerie, and Paula, each of you know what you mean to me and how much I appreciate the difference we make together. Thank you for always staying true to the message and leading the way, right by my side. And a special thanks to Paula Lippert. Your commitment to what's true and passion to make the world a better place inspire me.

Venice Nutrition and 8 Week Run community members, coaches, and partners—This book belongs to all of us, and the difference we make grows stronger by the day. Thank you for being part of this community and choosing to lead by example. Your actions are the motivational fuel so many people need to take their first step. This is truly just the beginning, and each of you forever have my appreciation.

About the Author

Most important, Mark Macdonald is a husband to his wife, Abbi, and father to their ten-year-old son, Hunter, and new baby girl, Hope. Professionally, he's a world-renowned nutrition and fitness expert, best-selling author, television personality, international teacher and speaker, and entrepreneur who has coached everyone from celebrities to athletes to business executives to busy moms on how to permanently improve their inner and outer health with proper nutrition, fitness, and lifestyle habits.

Mark is the founder of Venice Nutrition and the IBNFC: International Board of Nutrition and Fitness Coaching, author of the *New York Times* bestseller *Body Confidence,* the go-to health expert for both CNN and HLN, and co-host of the Daily Share segment "Transformation Tuesdays" on HLN.

Mark opened the first Venice Nutrition Consulting Center in Venice Beach, California, over fifteen years ago and it has since developed into a network of more than five hundred centers across the United States, Canada, and Europe. Mark is continually featured on national media and is the keynote speaker at events throughout the world, as well as leading live interactive webinars and videocasts.

To receive cutting-edge nutrition and fitness strategies, experience one of his in-person or online events, or find out more about Mark, please visit www.MarkMacdonald.TV.

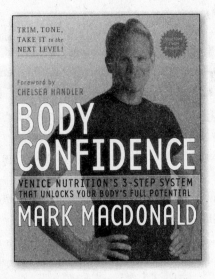
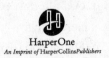